Clinical Cases for MRCPCH Applied Knowledge in Practice

July 2016

⋆RCPCH

**Royal College of
Paediatrics and Child Health**

Leading the way in Children's Health

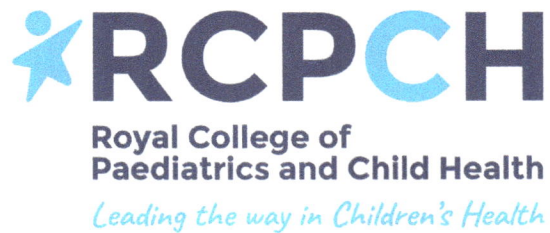

Editor
Dr Robert Dinwiddie

Deputy Editors
Dr Will Carroll
Dr Rob Primhak

Foreword by
Professor Neena Modi
President, Royal College of Paediatrics and Child Health

Foreword

The aim of this new textbook from the UK Royal College of Paediatrics and Child Health is to assist candidates to make sound clinical judgements based not on learning by rote, but through application of fundamental principles and an understanding of the underpinning science. The authors and editors are to be congratulated for producing an excellent, up-to-date resource.

Working through a diagnostic conundrum, from presentation, through careful history taking, and examination, supplemented by relevant investigations, is an intellectual challenge, a form of hypothesis testing, the goal of which is to arrive at a strong probability that the null hypothesis you have formulated should be rejected. Of course, the great privilege and responsibility of medicine, is that this isn't a game - your patients are counting on you getting it right!

This textbook will stand you in good stead for the MRCPH examinations, but above all, I hope you will enjoy dipping into it again and again.

Professor Neena Modi

President Royal College of Paediatrics and Child Health

Preface

The aim of the Applied Knowledge in Practice questions used in this part of the MRCPCH theory examinations is to test the candidate's ability to convert theoretical knowledge into practice by making appropriate clinical judgements based on the presentation and physical findings of commonly occurring case scenarios that are likely to be seen in everyday work.

The purpose of this book is to provide potential candidates with a series of clinically based questions identical in format to those that are used in the current computer-based exam. Every effort has been made to give as broad a view as possible of the type of clinical scenarios likely to be encountered. The cases described are also designed to cover all the subject headings included in the most recently updated syllabus available on the Royal College of Paediatrics and Child Health (RCPCH) website (1). Sample papers are also available on this website.

This volume builds on the scientific background comprehensively reviewed in the book Questions for the MRCPCH Theory and Science, which was published by the RCPCH in 2014. The aim of the discussion in each chapter here is to develop clinical knowledge from a research base into best practice for patient care.

Each chapter is based on a typical clinical scenario, followed by questions relevant to the topic. A succinct review of the subject is then given, interspersed with carefully chosen references relevant to the topic under discussion. These should also act as suggestions for further reading.

The best way to use this book is not to read it from cover to cover all at once. Each chapter should be reviewed individually by reading the case history, attempting the questions and learning from the accompanying discussion of the relevant subject. This can be done individually or in group sessions with other colleagues.

A significant number of consultants and senior trainees, all of whom have experience in this part of the theory examinations, have spent a great deal of time and effort in putting this together. Their work is highly appreciated, and it is hoped that readers will find that their contributions are a significant teaching aid as they prepare for this part of the exam.

A huge thank you is therefore due to my co-editors and the many chapter authors for their enthusiasm, patience, time and hard work in sharing their extensive personal experience and knowledge, especially for potential candidates at this level of training. Also, a special thank you is due to Sheran Mahal, the RCPCH administrator, who has spent a large amount of time and effort in putting this all together and bringing this important project to a successful conclusion.

Further acknowledgement must also be given to the many children and their parents who have allowed their "real-life" cases to be used in this book. Particular thanks is given to those who have granted permission for their clinical photographs to be used in this important context.

Similar tribute must also be paid to the spouses, partners and families of the question writers who have given of their precious "family time" together to allow for all the work required for this book to be put into place.

Dr Robert Dinwiddie

Vice Chair Applied Knowledge in Practice Examinations Board

1. www.rcpch.ac.uk Training, Examination and Professional Development. Updates – Examinations. Theory examinations. Structure and syllabi. Sample papers.

Contents

Chapter 1: A young person who harms themselves
Dr Karen Aucott, Dr Damian Wood

(1)

Sarah, a 15 year old girl, is brought to the emergency department after telling a teacher that she had taken paracetamol 3 hours earlier after an argument with her boyfriend. She cannot remember how many, but thinks it was most of the packet.

On arrival, she is quiet and withdrawn. She is reluctant to engage with the doctors in the emergency department but, on examination, they notice superficial lacerations to both forearms. She tells the nurse that she cuts herself when she is stressed but doesn't want her mother to know about it. She has been doing this for a while, but this is the first time she has ever been admitted to hospital. Paracetamol and salicylate levels are undetectable.

Q1. Which of the following would be the most appropriate action to take?

Select <u>one</u> answer only

A.   Admit her to a side room for privacy, given her emotional distress
B.   Admit her to the hospital for a psychosocial assessment within 24 hours
C.   Defer an assessment of safeguarding risks until the following day
D.   Discharge her home with a referral to child and adolescent mental health services (CAMHS)
E.   Inform the young person of the risks of injuring themselves

Q2. Which of the following is most likely to suggest an increased risk of true suicidal intent?

Select <u>one</u> answer only

A.   Being a smoker
B.   Having taken more than 30 paracetamol tablets
C.   Overdose was planned and she had left messages for friends and family
D.   Parental separation
E.   Presence of cutting to forearms

Answers and Rationale

Q1.   B: Admit her to the hospital for a psychosocial assessment within 24 hours
Q2.   C: Overdose was planned and she had left messages for friends and family

The topic area of child and adolescent mental health forms an important part of the syllabus for the Applied Knowledge paper (see 'syllabus mapping' below). Self-harm is defined as any form of behaviour that leads to self-injury, including cutting, burning, overdosing on medicines, preventing wound healing or hanging. Often the behaviour is a way of reducing emotional pain and distracting the young person from suicidal thoughts. It is important to consider the language used when discussing self-harm with adolescents; the young person should not feel judged regarding their behaviour and their emotional distress needs to be recognised and taken seriously. Self-harm is a serious public health problem and the rates of self-harm are a proxy indicator of the extent of mental health illness in young people within society (1). Approximately 25,000 adolescents present to hospitals in the UK each year following non-fatal self-harm, although it is estimated that only 1 in 10 children who do self-harm are seen by hospital services (1).

The first question is nuanced, and typifies some of the difficulties with the Applied Knowledge paper, and, indeed, some of those encountered as a more senior paediatrician. The knowledge that this young woman has undetectable paracetamol levels makes this question more testing. In deciding the best course of action it is helpful to consider which options would be unsafe. It would not be appropriate or safe to admit this patient to a side room until a full risk assessment of suicidal intention has been completed, as the patient needs to be easily observed at all times. A safeguarding assessment should take place at the time of admission, as this adds to the initial risk assessment; safeguarding issues may also be an underlying reason for self-harm behaviours. An outpatient referral is generally not advisable, as a full risk assessment by CAMHS should be undertaken promptly to assess the risk of further self-harm and the risk of suicidal intent. Advice given now about the risks of injury or harm as a result of inappropriate paracetamol ingestion may make the situation worse.

The second question requires an understanding of the evidence base concerning self-harm in young adults. Premeditated, rather than impulsive, self-harm is suggested by planning and consideration for events after death, and is an indicator for increased risk of true suicidal intent. There is no evidence to support a link between the number of tablets taken and the degree of suicidal intent. Similarly, evidence of other self-harm behaviour, such as cutting (also see below) does not help stratify suicidal intent. While parental separation may be a reason for emotional distress and self-harm behaviours, it does not have a direct link to suicidal intent. There is an association between mental health difficulties and premature death linked to risk behaviours such as smoking and alcohol, but it does not clearly inform suicide risk.

Adolescents may present to the emergency department with a range of self-harm thoughts or behaviours. These would range from discussing such thoughts through to completed suicide. Patients may appear aggressive or passive, agitated or withdrawn, and may express fear, anxiety or remorse. Most young people who self-harm do not have suicidal intent, but it is difficult to ascertain this at presentation when levels of distress are high. Cutting is the most common form of self-harm and is often impulsive. It usually indicates a maladaptation of the coping mechanism aimed at reducing emotional distress or anxiety. Girls are more likely to attempt self-harm than boys, but boys are at higher risk of completed suicide.

When assessing a person who presents with self-harm, it is important to consider the level of planning and intent, and the frequency of thoughts and actions that relate to self-harm or suicide. Other symptoms or signs that might suggest the presence of an underlying mental health illness are relevant, and would include a history of substance abuse and self-harm or suicidal behaviour in family members or the peer group.

It is helpful to consider the 4 Ps when assessing the patient: **predisposing** factors, **precipitating** factors, **perpetuating** or maintaining factors, and **protective** factors or resilience.

Psychosocial assessments such as the HEADSSS framework can be used to encourage adolescents to discuss difficulties. This structured assessment starts by asking simple questions about the young person's home life, education and activities before moving on to more sensitive topics such as drugs and alcohol, sex and relationships, self-harm behaviours and safety (2). In any such discussion with the young person, it is usually more helpful to focus on how the young person is feeling and what led to the self-harm behaviour rather than what the behaviour is itself.

Examples of safeguarding issues that might be revealed during a psychosocial assessment for self-harm include a young person who is worried she is pregnant, who may be the subject of child sexual exploitation, or who may have been raped. A much older 'partner' should always lead to more detailed enquiries. The possibility of a safeguarding risk should be seriously considered if a young person presents to the emergency department without a responsible adult, or if a parent or carer has not shown concern for the whereabouts of the young person.

There are recognised risk factors for suicidal behaviours, and these include depression and coexisting mental health issues such as anxiety. Previous suicide attempts, the use of drugs or alcohol when upset, and detailed planning on how to avoid discovery after the suicide attempt are all indicators of the risk of completed suicide or repetition of self-harm. A history of a relative or friend having committed suicide recently should be taken seriously. There has been relatively little research into factors that are protective against suicidal ideation and intent, but enhancing social skills, problem-solving abilities and the capacity of family and carers to offer emotional support are thought to be beneficial.

The care and management of young people who present with self-harm involves addressing any immediate medical needs, such as the treatment of the drug overdose to minimise any adverse effect. The medical management of a paracetamol overdose is a common topic in both the Foundation of Practice and Theory and Science examinations. The care and safety of the young person is paramount, and it is usual practice to admit them for a more detailed psychosocial assessment by adolescent mental health professionals. This must take place promptly while the young person is in hospital. The young person should be cared for on an open ward in view of the nursing staff so that safety can be monitored. Ongoing management is targeted towards addressing the underlying difficulties of the young person. It is important to ensure that they are given alternative mechanisms for coping with the pressures that make them consider self-harm.

Syllabus Mapping

Adolescent Health/Medicine

- Know how to assess and diagnose risk taking behaviours including non-adherence, self-harm, alcohol and substance misuse and make appropriate referral to specialist services

Behavioural Medicine/Psychiatry

- Understand the role of Child and Adolescent Mental Health Services (CAMHS) and know how to refer appropriately

References

1. eLFH.org, Adolescent Health Programme, Module 10: Self-harm and Common Mental Health Problems, http://e-lfh.org.uk

2. Klein DA, Goldenring JM, Adelman WP. HEEADSSS 3.0: The psychosocial interview for adolescents updated for a new century fuelled by media. http://contemporarypediatrics.modernmedicine.com/contemporary-pediatrics/content/tags/adolescent-medicine/heeadsss-30-psychosocial-interview-adolescence

Further Reading

Spender Q. Assessment of adolescent self-harm. Paediatrics and Child Health 2007; 17(11): 443–447.

NICE guidelines (CG16). Self-harm in over 8s: Short-term management and prevention of recurrence, Jul 2004, https://www.nice.org.uk/guidance/cg16.

NICE guidelines (CG133). Self-harm in over 8s: Long-term management, Nov 2011, https://www.nice.org.uk/guidance/cg133.

Chapter 2: A 15 month old with a cough and TB contact
Dr Lucy Hinds

(2)

A 15 month old boy has a 3 week history of cough. He was born in Slovakia and received a Bacille Calmette-Guérin (BCG) vaccination at birth. His maternal grandfather, who lives with the family, is receiving treatment for smear-positive pulmonary tuberculosis (TB). The boy's chest radiograph is normal and he has completed a week's course of amoxicillin. A Mantoux (tuberculin PPD) test is performed and, when read at 72 hours, there is a wheal measuring 16 mm in diameter.

Q1. Which investigation would be the most helpful at this point?

Select <u>one</u> answer only

A. Bronchoalveolar lavage
B. CT scan of the chest
C. Galactomannan
D. Gastric washings
E. Interferon gamma release assay (IGRA)

Q2. Which of the following statements about the BCG vaccine is correct?

Select <u>one</u> answer only

A. A single dose provides lifelong protection
B. It is a live attenuated vaccine
C. It provides greater protection from pulmonary than extra-pulmonary TB
D. It provides greater than 90% protection to vaccinated individuals
E. It transiently results in positive IGRA results

Q3. What is the best advice to give to parents of an infant with a 16 mm Mantoux test?

Select <u>one</u> answer only

A. Further testing is required to decide if this represents a mycobacterial infection
B. The results suggest an immunodeficiency and HIV testing is required
C. The young age makes a false positive result more likely
D. This is most likely to be the result of previous BCG
E. Treatment will be required

Answers and Rationale

Q1.   **D: Gastric washings**
Q2.   **B: It is a live attenuated vaccine**
Q3.   **E: Treatment will be required**

The history of contact with TB, along with the positive Mantoux test, makes the possibility of TB infection very likely. Despite the normal chest radiograph, it is possible that this child has active TB. The most useful investigation would be to send gastric washings on 3 consecutive mornings for microscopy for acid and alkaline fast bacilli (AAFB) and a culture of the Mycobacterium tuberculosis, in order to confirm a microbiological diagnosis of TB infection.

The key point in this case is to differentiate between latent and active TB infection, as this will determine the type and duration of treatment given. The UK NICE guidelines on the treatment of TB published in 2011 suggest that children aged between 4 weeks and 2 years who have been in close contact with smear-positive pulmonary TB should have a Mantoux test or tuberculin skin test (TST) (1).

Table 2.1: Interpretation of TST reaction

Induration of >5 mm is considered positive in:	Induration of >10 mm is considered positive in:	Induration of >15 mm is considered positive in:
HIV-infected individuals A recent contact of an individual with TB disease Individuals with fibrotic changes on chest radiograph consistent with previous TB infection Patients who have undergone organ transplants Individuals who are immunosuppressed for other reasons (e.g. taking the equivalent of >15 mg/day of prednisone for 1 month or longer, or taking TNF-α antagonists)	Recent immigrants (<5 years) from high-prevalence countries Intravenous drug users Residents and employees of high-risk congregate settings, e.g. detention facilities/refugee camps Mycobacteriology laboratory personnel Individuals with clinical conditions that place them at high risk Children <4 years of age Infants, children, and adolescents exposed to adults in high-risk categories	Any individual, including persons with no known risk factors for TB, including those with previous BCG vaccination

False-positive TSTs can result from contact with nontuberculous mycobacteria or vaccination with BCG, because the TST test material contains antigens that are also in BCG and certain nontuberculous mycobacteria. False positive results may also be due to the incorrect administration of TST or an incorrect interpretation of the test.

False negative results can also occur due to the following reasons:

- Cutaneous anergy (the inability to react to skin tests because of a weakened immune system)
- Recent TB infection (within 8–10 weeks of exposure)
- Very old TB infection
- Very young age (less than 6 months old)
- Recent (less than 4 weeks) live-virus vaccination (e.g. measles)
- Overwhelming TB disease
- Some viral illnesses (e.g. measles and chicken pox)
- Incorrect method of TST administration
- Incorrect interpretation of the reaction, insufficient dose and inadvertent subcutaneous injection

If the TST is positive, the child should be assessed for an active TB infection. For a child who has previously received a BCG vaccination and has a TST result of less than 15 mm, the test should be repeated after 6 weeks, together with an IGRA.

Gastric washings are based on the premise that young children are generally unable to expectorate, instead swallowing sputum into the stomach. Early morning gastric washings taken prior to the child eating or drinking, from a nasogastric tube already in situ, enable swallowed sputum to be sampled. In children with pulmonary TB, gastric lavage is more sensitive than bronchoalveolar lavage for the isolation of Mycobacterium tuberculosis, so bronchoalveolar lavage is a less appropriate option (2).

A CT scan of the chest may be a useful investigation to determine the nature and extent of lung disease, in view of the history of prolonged cough with a normal chest x-ray. A chest x-ray has low sensitivity and specificity in the diagnosis of TB, as its interpretation is very subjective; thoracic CT may identify hilar or mediastinal adenopathy in children with a positive TST and a normal chest X ray (3). However, a detailed radiological assessment of TB is less helpful than a microbiological diagnosis in this case.

Galactomannan is a polysaccharide component of the cell wall of the aspergillus species and other fungi. The galactomannan assay is an enzyme-linked immunosorbent assay (ELISA) and is used as a non-invasive test to screen for invasive aspergillus. It is has no role in the diagnosis of a suspected TB infection.

IGRAs detect sensitisation to Mycobacterium tuberculosis by measuring interferon gamma (IFN-γ) release in response to antigens representing *Mycobacterium tuberculosis*. IGRAs cannot distinguish between latent infection and active TB disease, and should not be used for diagnosis of active TB, (which is a microbiological diagnosis). A positive IGRA result may not necessarily indicate active TB and a negative IGRA result may not rule out active TB (4).

IGRAs are not affected by the BCG vaccination status, and are therefore useful for the evaluation of a latent TB infection in BCG-vaccinated individuals. IGRAs also appear to be unaffected by most infections with environmental nontuberculous mycobacteria, which can cause false-positive TSTs, with the exception of *Mycobacterium marinum*, *Mycobacterium kansasii*, *Mycobacterium szulgai*, and *Mycobacterium flavescens* (5).

At best, BCG provides 70–80% protection to children in developed countries and significantly less to those in developing countries. It is a live attenuated vaccine that provides greater protection from extra-pulmonary TB than primary pulmonary TB. A single dose only provides protection for 10–15 years and not for life.

Syllabus Mapping

Infection, Immunology and Allergy

- Be able to assess, diagnose and manage infections acquired in the UK and overseas including TB, HIV and know when to refer.

Respiratory Medicine with ENT

- Be able to assess and manage chronic cough including arranging and interpreting investigations when appropriate.

References and Further Reading

1. https://www.nice.org.uk/guidance/cg117.

2. Abadco, DL, Steiner M. Gastric lavage is better than bronchoalveolar lavage for isolation of Mycobacterium tuberculosis in childhood pulmonary tuberculosis. Pediatric Infectious Disease Journal 1992; 11: 9.

3. Garrido JB et al. Usefulness of thoracic CT to diagnose tuberculosis disease in patients younger than 4 years of age. Pediatr Pulmonol 2012; 47(9): 895–902.

4. Nayak S, Acharyia B. Mantoux testing and its interpretation. Indian Dermatol Online J 2012; 3(1): 2–6.

5. Sester M et al. Interferon-γ release assays for the diagnosis of active tuberculosis: A systematic review and meta-analysis. Eur Respir J 2011; 37(1): 100–11.

Chapter 3: A 9 year old girl with status epilepticus
Dr Gopalakrishnan Venkatachalam, Dr Jaya Sujatha Gopal Kothandapani

3

A previously fit and healthy 9 year old Caucasian girl presents to the emergency department in status epilepticus. She is reported to have had paranoid behaviour, a low-grade temperature and vomiting for a few days prior to her presentation. She was born at term with congenital pulmonary valve stenosis that warranted balloon dilatation at 10 weeks of age with no subsequent sequelae.

She requires intubation and ventilation for 3 days, and is treated with a midazolam infusion and intravenous phenytoin for seizure control along with intravenous cefotaxime and aciclovir for suspected encephalitis. Following extubation, she displays signs and symptoms of encephalopathy, including an altered level of consciousness with associated changes in behaviour, mood, emotion, speech and movement. CSF analysis shows pleocytosis (red blood cells 10×10^6/l, white blood cells 18×10^6/l) with a negative PCR for bacteria and viruses and a slightly raised Mycoplasma pneumoniae specific IgM CFT titre (1:160). The infection screen shows an initial C-reactive protein of 7 mg/l, which increases to 116 mg/l on day 3 of admission. A 3-week course of clarithromycin is completed; however, she remains apyrexial throughout the admission.

The EEG on day 1 shows high voltage rhythmic slow wave activity with prominent spikes in the left parietal region, raising the possibility of an encephalopathy or structural epileptogenic lesion. The CT brain scan on day 1 shows compression of the posterior part of right lateral ventricle with a bulky internal capsule. The MR brain scan on day 1 shows a high signal in the right hippocampus.

The investigation for causes of her evolving encephalopathy reveals hypothyroidism (TSH >100 mU/l (0.3–4.5), fT4 8.6 pmol/l (11–24), fT3 4.7 pmol/l (3–9)) with positive anti-peroxidase antibodies (711 IU/l) and anti-thyroglobulin antibodies (560 IU/l). The remainder of the autoimmune screen, including anti-NMDA receptor and anti-voltage gated potassium channel antibodies (VGKC antibodies), is negative. An ultrasound of the neck is consistent with thyroiditis.

Q1. Which of the following is the most likely diagnosis?

Select <u>one</u> answer only

A. Hashimoto's encephalitis
B. Limbic encephalitis
C. Mycoplasma pneumoniae encephalitis
D. Paraneoplastic encephalitis
E. Systemic lupus erythematosus

Q2. Which of the following would be the next line of management?

Select <u>one</u> answer only

A. Chemotherapy
B. IV immunoglobulin
C. Oral prednisolone
D. Serial plasma exchange for a year
E. Thyroidectomy

Answers and Rationale

Q1. A: Hashimoto's encephalitis
Q2: B: IV immunoglobulin

Encephalopathy

Reduced level of alertness/consciousness is the principal symptom/sign in encephalopathy. Many times, it may be preceded by headaches, vomiting, seizures and weakness or rash, depending on the aetiology. Assessing reduced consciousness accurately in infancy and in intellectually challenged children is neither simple nor easy. However, it is imperative to monitor the worsening or improvement of impairment of consciousness by an objective tool, the Glasgow Coma Scale score (1), which carries less inter-observer variability.

Table 3.1. Aetiology of encephalopthies

Infective
Autoimmune
Metabolic
Toxic substances
Epileptic encephalopathy (ictal and interictal epileptiform discharges that lead to cognitive, behavioural and motor regression)
Other systemic failures such uraemia and hepatic encephalopathy
Posterior reversible encephalopathy syndrome, secondary to hypertension and the use of immunosuppressants, e.g. tacrolimus, ciclosporin (rare).
Wernicke encephalopathy due to thiamine deficiency (rare)
Head injury

In general, investigating a child with encephalopathy should be specific and appropriate to the individual clinical presentation. Not all the investigations listed apply to all the patients.

Investigations:

Step 1:

Blood gas, U&Es, Liver function tests
Ammonia
CSF – Glucose and lactate paired with plasma
CSF – Microscopy, culture and sensitivity
Urine toxicology (if appropriate)

Step 2:

Neuroimaging – MRI brain scan (1.5 Tesla) and CT brain scan in suspected intracranial haemorrhage as first-line treatment
Metabolic screening: plasma and urine – Organic and amino acids, ketones

Thyroid profile
CSF – Oligoclonal bands, IgG index
Anti-neuronal antibodies

Step 3:

EEG/video telemetry
Heavy metal measurement, e.g. copper
Vitamin measurement, e.g. thiamine

Infective encephalitis

Infective encephalitis is generally due to direct invasion by viruses, bacteria, fungi or parasites. In the paediatric age group, the most common cause for encephalitis is Herpes simplex type 1 virus infection; however, Herpes simplex type 2 is common among immune-compromised individuals and neonates. Kneen *et al.* (2012) have proposed an algorithm to approach suspected viral encephalitis on behalf of the National Encephalitis Guidelines Development and Stakeholder Groups (2), which is easy and simple to use. All children who are suspected to have encephalitis should initially be treated with IV aciclovir and IV antibiotics until an infective cause has been ruled out.

Autoimmune encephalitis

Autoimmune encephalitis comes under the umbrella term of autoimmune central nervous system disorders, and this clinical entity evolves as a result of misdirected and upregulation of the patient's own immune system. Its pathological and clinical manifestations may be localised to 1 region in the brain, as seen in limbic encephalitis and basal ganglia encephalitis. It can also be a part of polyfocal involvement, such as in acute disseminated encephalomyelitis (ADEM). ADEM can present with a constellation of symptoms and signs, such as mood disorders, ataxia, pyramidal tract deficit, movement disorder and seizures, with significant multiple high signal changes in MRI brain imaging (3).

The mainstay of treatment is based on immune modulation by intravenous corticosteroids, immunoglobulin and plasma exchange with or without immunosuppressant therapy, depending on the severity and responsiveness of the condition.

Metabolic encephalopathy

These are a heterogeneous group of inborn errors of metabolism (IEM) disorders, which include amino acid and organic acid disorders, urea cycle defects and mitochondrial disorders. These can present with a myriad of symptoms and signs, such as encephalopathy, seizures, visual disturbances, stroke-like episodes, headaches, hypotonia, ptosis, ophthalmoplegia, ataxia, myoclonus and bulbar palsy. Suspecting a metabolic disorder is a first step and pivotal in the process of diagnosing IEMs. In particular, mitochondrial disorders can manifest in any organ and often mimic other, more recognisable, disorders (4).

In many IEMs, the management is mainly focused on symptom-based treatment and other supportive therapy. On the other hand, some of the IEMs respond to specific vitamins and co-factors treatment, e.g. thiamine, riboflavin, co-enzyme Q10 and carnitine. It is essential to know that some medications, such as sodium valproate or aspirin, can lead to metabolic decompensation in selected conditions. Prenatal diagnosis and genetic counselling have to be a part of comprehensive management.

Posterior reversible encephalopathy syndrome (PRES)

This is a rare type of encephalopathy that can present with altered mental status, headaches, vomiting, seizures and visual disturbances. It is mainly associated with systemic hypertension, and is also rarely seen in immunosuppressive therapy (chemotherapy). An MRI brain scan with diffusion-weighted images would be the best method to distinguish PRES from other types of encephalopathy. Treatment consists of controlling blood pressure, eliminating the causative drugs, and supportive management (5, 6).

Hashimoto's encephalopathy

This rare relapsing encephalopathy presents specifically with neuropsychiatric features, seizures and neurologic deficits. It is associated with high serum anti-thyroid antibodies with or without hypothyroidism (7, 8). Immune modulation may be recommended depending on the severity of the disease process and its manifestations. Children with Hashimoto's disease need long-term monitoring.

Syllabus Mapping

Neurology

- Know the indications for and limitations of neurophysiological studies e.g. EEG, EMG, BAER, otoacoustic emissions and be able to recognise abnormal EEG patterns.

- Be able to assess, diagnose and manage acute infections of the nervous system

- Be able to assess diagnose and manage seizure disorders and conditions which may mimic them.

References and Further Reading

1. Teasdale G, Maas A, Lecky F et al. The Glasgow Coma Scale at 40 years: Standing the test of time. Lancet Neurology 2014; 13: 844–854.

2. Kneen R, Michael BD, Menson D et al. Management of suspected viral encephalitis in children – Association of British Neurologists and British Paediatric Allergy, Immunology and Infection Group National Guidelines. Journal of Infection 2012: 64: 449–477.

3. Idrissovaa ZhR, Boldyrevab MN, Dekonenkoco EP et al. Acute disseminated encephalomyelitis in children: Clinical features and HLA-DR linkage. European Journal of Neurology 2003; 10: 537–546.

4. Koenig MK. Presentation and Diagnosis of Mitochondrial Disorders in Children. Pediatr Neurol 2008; 38: 305–313.

5. Chen TH, Lin WC, Tseng YH et al. Posterior Reversible Encephalopathy in Children – Case Series and Systematic Review. J Child Neurol 2013; 28: 1378–1386.

6. Morris EB, Laningham FH, Sandlund JT, Raja B, Khan RB. Posterior Reversible Encephalopathy Syndrome in Children with Cancer. Pediatr Blood Cancer 2007; 48: 152–159.

7. Erol I, Saygi S, Alehan F. Hashimoto's encephalopathy in children and adolescents. Pediatr Neurol 2011; 45: 420–422.

8. Mamoudjy NI, Korff C, Maurey H et al. Hashimoto's encephalopathy: Identification and long-term outcome in children. Eur J Paediatr 2013; 17: 280–287.

Chapter 4: An 11 year old girl with seizures
Dr Gopalakrishnan Venkatachalam

(4)

Amy is an 11 year old girl who is known to have drug resistant epilepsy. She attends the epilepsy clinic with her mother, who is worried about the recent worsening of her tonic seizures. She had her first seizure when she was 7 months old. This consisted of epileptic spasms and her EEG at that time showed hypsarrhythmia. She responded well to prednisolone therapy and remained seizure free for a year. When she was 2 years old, she again developed epileptic spasms that did not respond to anti-epileptic drugs (AEDs) and, at 3 years of age, she was diagnosed as having refractory epilepsy.

Now aged 11 years, she suffers from multiple seizure types including tonic seizures, absence seizures, myoclonic seizures and generalised tonic-clonic seizures. She is being treated with various AEDs and a ketogenic diet, none of which are able to control her seizures. Currently, she is taking optimum doses of phenytoin, levetiracetam and clobazam. She is also receiving vitamin D supplements due to vitamin D deficiency. Her recent history also suggests that, over the last few years, she has regressed in her cognitive skills.

The physical examination shows that she has nystagmus and ataxia. During the examination, she has a tonic drop attack. No asymmetrical neurological signs are found and there is no evidence of raised intracranial pressure. Systemic examination of her heart, chest and abdomen is unremarkable.

Q1. Which of the following is the most likely diagnosis?

Select <u>one</u> answer only

A.   Dravet syndrome
B.   Landau-Kleffner syndrome
C.   Lennox-Gastaut syndrome
D.   Progressive myoclonic epilepsy
E.   West syndrome

Q2. Which of the following is the most important next test to perform?

Select <u>one</u> answer only

A.   EEG
B.   Invasive intracranial pressure monitoring
C.   Ketone levels
D.   MRI brain scan
E.   Phenytoin level

Q3. Which of the following is the next most appropriate for the long-term treatment of her increased tonic seizures?

Select <u>one</u> answer only

A.   Deep Brain Stimulation (DBS)
B.   Frontal lobectomy
C.   Increase the dose of her AEDs
D.   Ketogenic diet
E.   Vagal Nerve Stimulation (VNS)

Answers and Rationale

Q1.   **C: Lennox-Gastaut syndrome**
Q2.   **E: Phenytoin level**
Q3.   **E: Vagal Nerve Stimulation (VNS)**

Epilepsy

Epilepsy is one of the debilitating neurological conditions that can start at any age – from infancy (such as in West syndrome) to adulthood (such as in post-traumatic or post-operative epilepsy). In the paediatric population, epilepsy has varying degrees of impact on the patient's physical and psychosocial wellbeing and, as a consequence, it also may affect their neurodevelopment.

Every individual has some risk of developing a seizure in their lifetime. A seizure can be defined as a clinical manifestation of an abnormal excessive hypersynchronous discharge of a group of cortical neurons. Recently, the definition of epilepsy has been modified by the International League Against Epilepsy (ILAE) task force as 2 unprovoked seizures occurring more than 24 hours apart or 1 unprovoked seizure with more than a 60% risk of developing another seizure over 10 years (1).

Based on the aetiology, epilepsy is classified into 3 major groups: genetic (epilepsy as a direct result of a known or presumed genetic defect), structural/metabolic, and unknown (where the nature of underlying cause is unknown). The terms 'idiopathic' and 'cryptogenic' are now obsolete (2). A special group or category called epileptic encephalopathy is a heterogeneous group of epilepsies where ictal and interictal epileptiform discharges lead to cognitive, behavioural and motor regression (3).

Table 4.1: Epilepsy syndromes/encephalopathies based on the age of onset

Neonatal onset	Early myoclonic encephalopathy
	Ohtahara syndrome
Infantile onset	West syndrome
	Dravet syndrome
Childhood onset	Landau-Kleffner syndrome
	Lennox-Gastaut syndrome

Investigations

AED treatment is not without side effects; hence, it is absolutely essential to warn patients and parents about this, as well as to look for side effects in the follow-up clinic – for example, rash due to lamotrigine, weight gain due to sodium valproate and word finding (language) difficulties due to topiramate. Drug-to-drug interactions with AEDs are also quite common, especially with lamotrigine and sodium valproate. These interactions influence the drug levels in the blood, which warrants monitoring their measurement and adjusting the dose accordingly. Otherwise, checking AED levels regularly is not required but is a useful tool when there is an upsurge of seizure frequency, evidence of drug toxicity, or concerns about the patient's adherence to treatment.

A phenytoin level is likely to be helpful in this child, as it may give an indication of overall adherence as well as determining whether there is scope for an adjustment to the dosing. It is simple to perform and relatively easy to interpret and should be considered in preference to the other options.

An EEG would be a first-line investigation in epilepsy; however, on many occasions, it is neither a diagnostic nor a confirmative test except in conditions such as absence seizures and infantile spasms. In general, an EEG has a low sensitivity (25–56%) with better specificity (78–98%) (4). Epileptiform discharges can occur without having an epileptic seizure. Abnormal epileptiform discharges have been seen in 2–4% of healthy children on routine EEGs. To improve the yield, the EEG can be recorded during wakefulness and sleep. It can also be augmented by hyperventilation and photic stimulation.

A scalp EEG has its own limitations, as it records electrical discharges from the surface of the scalp with significant artefacts related to facial muscle movements. Invasive EEG – electrocorticography (ECoG) – measures electrical signals directly over the surface of the brain itself; this is more accurate, with the near absence of artefacts. It is, however, an invasive procedure that requires neurosurgery to implant the EEG leads onto the surface of the brain, with its own risks and complications.

The next level of investigation would be neuroimaging, including MRI and other functional MRIs, such as positron emission tomography (PET) and single photon emission computed tomography (SPECT). When epilepsy secondary to metabolic disease is suspected, CSF analysis for specific disorders is indicated. Examples would include CSF lactate in mitochondrial disorders, CSF glucose in GLUT-1 disorder, and CSF amino acids and neurotransmitters when necessary.

In general, a significant proportion of epileptic disorders respond to the currently available pharmacological treatments. However, 30–40% of epilepsies are drug resistant. Drug resistant epilepsy has been defined as the failure of adequate trials of 2 tolerated and appropriately chosen and used AED schedules (whether as monotherapies or in combination) to achieve sustained seizure freedom. Predictive factors of drug resistance include age of onset, multiple seizure types and associated cerebral lesions (5, 6).

Non-pharmacological treatments of epilepsy

A ketogenic diet, low carbohydrate and high fat containing diets increase ketosis with high blood ketone levels, which, in turn, attenuates spontaneous firing in the neurons. As a result, this can cause short- to medium-term benefits in seizure control (7). VNS is an add-on treatment for refractory epilepsy. VNS comprises of a battery-operated generator that is connected to the left vagal nerve by a wire, and a magnetic wand. It has been used successfully in children to reduce the frequency of tonic and atonic drop seizures (8). It is not without side effects, e.g. cough and hoarseness of voice (8, 9). Epilepsy surgery is another novel alternative treatment for focal onset drug resistant epilepsy. Depending on the type and location of the brain lesion, the epilepsy surgeon chooses the type of the surgery required (lesionectomy, lobectomy, callosotomy or hemispherectomy). Selecting the right patient for the specific type of surgery involved can offer the patient good seizure control (10).

Syllabus Mapping

Neurology

- Know the indications for and limitations of neurophysiological studies e.g. EEG, EMG, BAER, otoacoustic emissions and be able to recognise common EEG patterns.

- Be able to assess, diagnose and manage seizure disorders and conditions which my may mimic them.

References and Further Reading

1. Fisher RS, Acevedo C, Arzimanoglou A et al. A practical definition of epilepsy. Epilepsia 2014; 55: 475–482.

2. Berg AT, Scheffer IE. New concepts in classification of the epilepsies: Entering the 21st century. Epilepsia 2011; 52: 1058–1062.

3. Covanis A. Epileptic encephalopathies (including severe epilepsy syndromes). Epilepsia 2012; 53(Suppl. 4): 114–126.

4. Smith SJM. EEG in the diagnosis, classification, and management of patients with epilepsy. J Neurol Neurosurg Psychiatry 2005; 76: ii2–ii7. doi: 10.1136/jnnp.2005.069245

5. Russo A, Posar A, Conti S, Parmeggiani A. [Epub ahead of print] Prognostic factors of drug resistant epilepsy in childhood, an Italian study. Pediatr Int 2015. doi: 10.1111/ped.12705

6. Kwan P, Arzimanoglou A, Berg AT et al. Definition of drug-resistant epilepsy: Consensus proposal by the ad hoc task force of the ILAE Commission on Therapeutic Strategies. Epilepsia 2010; 51: 1069–77.

7. Levy RG, Cooper PN, Giri P. Ketogenic diet and other dietary treatments for epilepsy. Cochrane Database Syst Rev 2012; 3: CD001903. doi: 10.1002/14651858.CD001903.pub2

8. Rosenfeld WE, Roberts DW. Tonic and atonic seizures: What's next – VNS or callosotomy? Epilepsia 2009; 50(Suppl 8): 25–30.

9. Lulic D, Ahmadian A, Baaj AA, Benbadis SR, Vale FL. Vagus nerve stimulation. Neurosurg Focus 200; 27(3): E5. doi: 10.3171/2009.6.FOCUS09126

10. Téllez-Zenteno JF, Dhar R, Hernandez-Ronquillo L, Wiebe S. Long-term outcomes in epilepsy surgery: Antiepileptic drugs, mortality, cognitive and psychosocial aspects. Brain 2007; 130: 334–45.

Chapter 5: A 1 year old with fever and an abnormal blood result
Dr Poothirikovil Venugopalan

5

A 1 year old Caucasian boy presents to the emergency department with fever, vomiting and a skin rash of 2 days' duration. Examination suggests a viral illness. However, in view of the rash with fever, he has blood investigations.

Investigations

Blood

Haemoglobin	90 g/l	
White cell count	10×10^9/l	
Platelets	400×10^9/l	
MCV	70 fl (77–91)	
MCH	20 pg (23–31)	
MCHC	28 g/dl (32–35)	
Reticulocyte count	20×10^9/l (25–100)	
Ferritin	42 µmol/l (41–400	
Sodium	139 mmol/l	
Potassium	5.2 mmol/l	
Urea	3.3 mmol/l	
Creatinine	30 mmol/l	
CRP	20 mg/l	

Q1. Which of the following is the most likely cause of the low haemoglobin?

Select <u>one</u> answer only

A.   Acute leukaemia
B.   Anaemia secondary to blood loss
C.   Anaemia secondary to infection
D.   Haemoglobinopathy
E.   Iron deficiency anaemia

Q2. Which of the following will confirm the diagnosis?

Select <u>one</u> answer only

A.   Bone marrow aspiration
B.   Liver function tests
C.   Repeat serum ferritin in 2 weeks
D.   Stool for occult blood
E.   Thyroid function tests

Answer and Rationale

Q1. **E: Iron deficiency anaemia**
Q2. **C: Repeat serum ferritin in 2 weeks**

Here are the blood results with normal values in brackets:

Haemoglobin	90 g/l (110–140)
White cell count	10 x 10⁹/l (5–12)
Platelets	400 x 10⁹/l (150–450)
MCV	70 fl (77–91)
MCH	20 pg (23–31)
MCHC	28 g/dl (32–35)
Reticulocyte count	20 x 10⁹/l (25–100)
Ferritin	42 µg/l (41–400)
Sodium	139 mmol/l (133–146)
Potassium	5.2 mmol/l (3.5–5.5)
Urea	3.3 mmol/l (2.5–6.5)
Creatinine	30 µmol/l (13–39)
CRP	20 mg/l (<10)

These results support the clinical diagnosis of a viral illness. However, this child also has anaemia with low MCV, MCH, and MCHC. All these are suggestive of iron deficiency anaemia. The reticulocyte count is low, also supporting the diagnosis.

The history is not consistent with leukaemia, and the platelet count is normal. Haemoglobinopathies can show similar blood results, but are rare in Caucasians, and the serum ferritin can be high (rather than near the lower end of the range as in this child). Anaemia secondary to infection is usually a normocytic, normochromic anaemia. There is no history of blood loss in this child, and the platelet count is normal (a high platelet count, when present, may indicate ongoing occult blood loss).

Serum ferritin is a non-specific inflammatory marker, and can be elevated in the presence of any systemic infection, including viral illnesses. So the near normal serum ferritin value in this child does not preclude the diagnosis of iron deficiency.

The most common cause of a microcytic, hypochromic anaemia is iron deficiency, generally secondary to the poor dietary intake of iron (Box 5.1). However, malabsorption (as in coeliac disease) can present similarly; hence, it would be advisable to arrange a blood test for a coeliac screen for this child. Any source of occult blood loss also needs to be excluded by a urine dipstick and stool examination for occult blood.

Box 5.1: Causes of microcytic anaemia in infancy

Iron deficiency anaemia:

Deficient intake, e.g. nutritional anaemia
Defective absorption, e.g. coeliac disease
Increased loss, e.g. cow's milk intolerance

Anaemia of chronic disease
Thalassaemia
Sideroblastic anaemia

Iron deficiency is one of the most prevalent nutrient deficiencies in infancy and early childhood (1). At birth and during early infancy, the haemoglobin level falls and the iron content of the body is sufficient to meet the ongoing requirements. However, by the age of 4 months, neonatal iron stores are reduced by half, and exogenous iron is required to maintain haemoglobin concentration during the rapid phase of growth between 4 and 12 months.

The early introduction of unmodified cow's milk as the major milk source at around 6 months of age is the most common dietary characteristic of infants found to have iron deficiency anaemia at 1 year. In the UK, iron deficiency is more common in those children consuming over 1 litre of cow's milk daily and in those in whom unmodified cow's milk was introduced before 8 months of age (2). Cow's milk is low in iron, but the existing evidence suggests that other causes, including weaning foods, when not adequate in iron content, are at least as important in causing iron deficiency. Deficiency of iron manifests initially as a fall in serum ferritin, and later on as a reduction in the haemoglobin concentration of the blood.

Most affected infants are asymptomatic. However, the deficiency can be associated with many systemic abnormalities: blue sclerae, koilonychia, impaired exercise capacity, and an increased susceptibility to infection. Abnormal developmental performance and poor growth have also been reported.

Once diagnosed, management consists of iron supplementation that is to be continued until at least 3 months after the haemoglobin level reaches the normal value for the age. Attention to the diet and advice on improvement (including sufficient iron containing foods) will help to sustain the benefit of iron therapy (Box 5.2).

Box 5.2: Foods rich in iron

- Apricots, prunes and raisins
- Beans and lentils
- Eggs
- Fish
- Leafy green vegetables
- Meat
- Oatmeal
- Tuna

Primary prevention can be achieved by ensuring sufficient dietary iron from 4 months of age and throughout the weaning period. This can be through giving supplementary iron, by the fortification of foods, and by dietary education that changes the feeding practice. Programmes for screening and treating affected infants and children are being proposed, but these have not yet received universal approval (3, 4).

Syllabus Mapping

Nutrition

- Be able to assess, diagnose and manage malnutrition, obesity and their complications

References and Further Reading

1. Lopez A, Cacoub P, MacDougall IC, Peyrin-Biroulet L. Iron deficiency anaemia. Lancet 2016; 387: 907-16.

2. Booth IW, Aukett MA. Iron deficiency anaemia in infancy and early childhood. Arch Dis Child 1997; 76: 549– 54.

3. World Health Organisation. Iron deficiency anaemia: Assessment, prevention and control. A guide for programme managers. http://www.who.int/nutrition/publications/en/ida_assessment_prevention_control.pdf.

4. Siu AL for US Preventive Services Task Force. Screening for Iron Deficiency Anemia in Young Children: USPSTF Recommendation Statement. Pediatrics 2015; 136: 746–52. doi: 10.1542/peds.2015-2567

Chapter 6: A 4 year old who requires palliative care analgesia
Dr Hannah King, Dr Martin Hewitt

6

A 4 year old boy with a stage IV neuroblastoma has relapsed for the second time after receiving treatment with systemic chemotherapy, surgical resection of the abdominal mass and radiotherapy to the abdominal site. He is currently an in-patient on the ward. All treatment options have been explored and, following long discussions with his parents, it has been decided that palliative care is now appropriate.

He has developed significant bone pain with a particular focus at the mid shaft of his right femur. A lytic lesion has been identified at that site. Over the last 24 hours, he has received 5 mg oral morphine solution at 02:10, 07:20, 12:00, 15:00, 19:50 and 23:30. However, he remains unsettled and in pain. You are asked to review his requirements for further analgesia.

Q1. Which of the following regimes would you prescribe for him now?

Select <u>one</u> answer only

A.   Continue with oral morphine 5 mg every 4 hours
B.   Oral morphine 5 mg every 3 hours
C.   Slow release morphine 5 mg twice daily (with oral morphine for breakthrough pain)
D.   Slow release morphine 15 mg twice daily (with oral morphine for breakthrough pain)
E.   Slow release morphine 20 mg twice daily (with oral morphine for breakthrough pain)

Q2. Which of the following is the most appropriate approach to his femoral pain if the above increased dosing does not help?

Select <u>one</u> answer only

A.   Epidural anaesthesia
B.   Further increase in oral morphine dose
C.   Intralesion steroids
D.   Local radiotherapy
E.   Spinal block

Answers and Rationale

Q1.   E: Slow release morphine 20 mg twice daily (with oral morphine for breakthrough pain)
Q2.   D: Local radiotherapy

The child remains in pain despite the previous 24 hours of regular oral morphine. In an attempt to improve pain control, it would be wise to change to a slow release preparation (1). The total amount given in the preceding 24 hours is calculated (30 mg in this case) and a new dose given which should be 25–30% greater than before (thus, 40 mg). This is then split between 2 dosing times. Analgesia for breakthrough pain must also be prescribed.

Local pain control must not create unwanted side effects that may cloud the palliative period. Epidural and spinal blocks would impact lower limb motor control, along with continence control. Increasing the dose of systemic analgesia at this point would produce generalised side effects. Intralesional steroids are rarely used, although they may work in conditions that are steroid-sensitive but not in neuroblastoma. Local radiotherapy will be effective.

The move to providing palliative care does not occur at a specific time point, but usually comes after a discussion with the patient – if old enough to understand the implications of such a discussion – and the family. These discussions will be difficult, but it is important to work with the patient and family members to understand their fears and wishes. An open and honest discussion will advise them that the options for a curative outcome have been exhausted, and the focus of care should move towards symptom control. This transition may take place over a long period of time in patients with chronic conditions. Such discussions, however difficult, will provide the opportunity to fulfil lifetime ambitions.

The importance of a clear, written record of any such conversations cannot be overstated, as this will form the basis of communication during the palliative period.

The symptoms that cause problems and difficulties are varied, and will depend upon the underlying clinical diagnosis and its location within the patient.

Pain is a common symptom and one that often causes concern with the patient and family members (2). It is important to ensure good pain control is maintained and plans are in place to respond quickly to escalating pain. During the early phases of palliative care, adequate pain control may be obtained with simple analgesics such as paracetamol or ibuprofen. The use of non-steroidal anti-inflammatory medication can be particularly useful for bone pain. Intermittent administration of analgesia is likely to become ineffective over time, and the use of analgesics on a regular and frequent basis should be the next step.

If pain is not controlled with regular and simple analgesics, it is usual to add oral opioid-based analgesics on a regular dosing regimen (3). Once pain is controlled and the total daily dose is established, then it is possible to convert to a slow release version and so provide more acceptable and consistent control.

The move to slow release medication must always be supported with oral morphine for breakthrough pain. It is usual to take the amount of opioid used in the previous 24 hours and give one sixth of this for each breakthrough dose. Dose escalation of the background medication may be necessary, and it is often considered appropriate to increase the daily dose by increments of 25–30%.

It is important to remember that changes between routes of administration require a dose adjustment, such as oral to IV morphine. There is no equivalence of doses in the different preparations. Changing between opiates (oral morphine to transdermal fentanyl patch) also requires a dose conversion and must only be undertaken after consulting a pharmacopoeia (1, 5).

Ketamine may have a role in those patients who have pain that is difficult to control by the above regime. The drug can be given orally or intravenously, and potentiates the effect of morphine. The oral route is associated with a peak-and-trough effect, and may result in hallucinations; this can limit its acceptability.

The introduction of opioid analgesic clearly brings with it the potential for unwanted side effects. The most common one is that of constipation, and it is therefore important to introduce a laxative to counter this side effect. Nausea and vomiting are also common and unpleasant side effects that must be anticipated and treated. Similarly, pruritus can be troublesome and ondansetron or cetirizine can be helpful.

Anxiety is commonly encountered and is often a cause for concern for the child and the family. Buccal or intravenous midazolam is effective; however, if the latter route is used, it is necessary to ensure that a supply of buccal medication is available for peaks of distress.

Another recognised and troublesome symptom is that of excess salivation. This is commonly seen in patients with tumours that affect the central nervous system, particularly those within the brainstem. Pharmacological options include the use of atropine-like agents, although they may convert copious loose secretions into reduced, but tenacious, secretions that are much more difficult to clear with suction.

Mobility difficulties can impact the value of the palliative period and require advice and input from physiotherapists and occupational therapists. Spiritual and psychological aspects for the patient and family need consideration, and this will again require the advice of the multidisciplinary team. An understanding of the requirements that surround death for differing faith groups is important in the provision of good palliative care.

Although direct care of the patient will end with their death, it is important to remember that family members may need support and advice for many years afterwards. Consequently, early contact and good communication with the local community teams is important (4).

Syllabus mapping

Palliative Care

- Understand and be able to apply pharmacological and non-pharmacological interventions in palliative care

References

1. BNF for Children 2015–2016:225-227. Pharmpress.com

2. Goldman A, Hewitt M, Collins GS, Childs M, Hain R. Symptoms in Children/Young People With Progressive Malignant Disease. Pediatrics 2006; 117: e1179–e1186.

3. Hewitt M, Goldman AA, Collins GS, Childs M, Hain R. Opioid use in palliative care of children and young people. J Pediatrics 2008; 152: 39–44.

4. Rebecca E, MacDonell-Yilmaz RE. Learning to care at the end. Pediatrics 2015; 135: 796–797.

5. Association for Paediatric Palliative Medicine Master Formulary 2012, 2nd edition. www.appm.org.uk.

Further Reading

Johnson LM, Snaman JM, Cupit MC, Baker JN. End-of-life care for hospitalised children. Pediatric Clinics of North America 2014; 61: 835–854.

Schwantes S, O'Brien HW. Pediatric palliative care for children with complex chronic medical conditions . Pediatric Clinics of North America 2014; 61: 797–821.

Hain R, Heckford E, McCulloch R. Paediatric palliative medicine in the UK: Past, present, future. Arch Dis Child 2012; 97: 381–384.

Singh JS. Basic Symptom Control in Paediatric Palliative Care: The Rainbows Children's Hospice Guidelines 2011, 8th edition. ACT (Association for Children's Palliative Care). www.togetherforshortlives. org.uk/professionals/resources/.

Chapter 7: A 15 year old girl with concerns about her weight

Dr Karen Aucott, Dr Damian Wood

7

Sophie is a 15 year old girl who is reviewed in an outpatient clinic as her parents have become concerned about her weight. She has always been active, competing in swimming at the national level, but has recently taken a keen interest in running as well. She has become more concerned about the types of food she eats and is insisting on coming home for lunch rather than having lunch with her friends. She has started missing meals and her schoolwork has deteriorated slightly. Her mood has changed, and she is described as 'unhappy' by her siblings. Her mother thinks she has gone down a dress size over the past 2 months.

On examination, she is thin with sunken cheeks and is cool peripherally with a central capillary refill time of 4 seconds. Her pulse is 55/minute and blood pressure 80/50 mmHg with orthostatic changes. Her body mass index (BMI) is 79% of the median BMI for her age. The rest of the examination is normal.

Q1. Which of the following additional features would support a diagnosis of anorexia nervosa?

Select <u>one</u> answer only

A.	Avoids reading food articles in magazines
B.	Feels others will avoid her if she gains weight
C.	Poor concentration and recall
D.	Pulse of 65/minute at rest
E.	Sleeps for long periods of time

A decision is made to admit Sophie to the ward.

Q2. What is the most appropriate step to reduce the risk of developing complications from refeeding?

Select <u>one</u> answer only

A.	Monitor serum electrolytes, calcium and phosphate daily
B.	Prescribe IV fluids
C.	Prescribe IV thiamine
D.	Request daily weights
E.	Start nasogastric feeding

Answers and Rationale

Q1.   **B: Feels others will avoid her if she gains weight**
Q2.   **A: Monitor serum electrolytes, calcium and phosphate daily**

Sophie has a diagnosis of anorexia nervosa. This diagnosis requires the presence of a persistent restriction of energy intake, leading to significantly low body weight. This process is coupled with an intense fear of gaining weight or of becoming fat, and the individual will demonstrate persistent behaviour that interferes with weight gain (even though the individual already has significantly low weight). There is a disturbance in the way the young person perceives their body weight or shape. Poor concentration and bradycardia are seen in patients with anorexia; however, such features are not required to make the diagnosis (1).

Sophie has a significant loss of weight and is at risk of developing refeeding syndrome (2). Monitoring of electrolytes, calcium and phosphate aims to biochemically detect refeeding syndrome before clinical symptoms manifest. Daily weights and rewards for weight gain are all counterproductive and will increase the anxiety levels that are already present. Antidepressants and nasogastric feeding are not first-line treatments. Intravenous fluids may precipitate overt cardiac failure.

Eating disorders in adolescents are associated with significant morbidity and mortality (3). The diagnosis should be considered when a young person presents with unhealthy practices around weight control, an abnormal preoccupation with body weight, size and shape, and recognised physical complications of an eating disorder. The disorder is egosyntonic (ideas and behaviours that fit with one's own image of self) and this may lead to ambivalence about recovery and even resistance to treatment.

The initial assessment of a patient with anorexia nervosa should focus on identifying the abnormal thinking about weight, body image and diet that are apparent to those close to the young person. It is also important to assess the potential physical complications of an eating disorder that include cardiac problems such as bradycardia, hypotension, orthostatic changes in blood pressure and heart rate, arrhythmias and prolonged QT identified on an electrocardiogram (ECG). Dry skin and lanugo hair may develop as the illness progresses. Pubertal arrest or delay is common, as is hypoglycaemia. The young person often complains of poor concentration, fatigue, muscle weakness and constipation. Liver and renal failure can occur in prolonged and severe malnutrition. At the first assessment, it is important to ensure that other causes of anorexia and weight loss – such as coeliac disease, endocrine disease, inflammatory bowel disease or malignancy – are ruled out.

Eating disorders are associated with other mental health comorbidities, including depression, anxiety and an obsessive-compulsive disorder. A psychosocial assessment (such as HEADSSS (4)) should be completed to help identify any trigger events or comorbidities.

The majority of patients can be treated in an outpatient setting. This involves a coordinated approach from a multidisciplinary team that includes child and adolescent mental health colleagues, dieticians and paediatricians. Initial treatment involves family-based therapy – an established psychological method that aims to empower parents to recognise the central role they have in changing a young person's behaviour. In some circumstances, it is more appropriate for a young person to be admitted, and this may be due to the severity of the disease, the presence of physical complications or the failure of outpatient treatment.

In parallel to the family-based therapy, there is a need for nutritional rehabilitation and weight restoration. An individualised meal plan should be introduced that aims to restore weight safely and steadily (generally 0.5 kg/week). The plan will also support the family in understanding the types and quantities of food needed to maintain this weight gain. In the majority of cases, oral feeding is the best option, as this allows the young person to physically experience the amount of food necessary for weight gain and helps to restore healthy eating behaviours.

Energy expenditure will also need to be balanced during weight restoration and, depending on the severity of illness; the amount of physical activity will be restricted to a minimum. Subsequent management aims to move the young person towards becoming more independent at managing their own eating, and ensuring that adolescent development progresses normally once a healthy weight has been reached.

When nutrition is reintroduced after a long period of starvation, there is a risk that the young person may develop the 'refeeding syndrome'. Although this is rare, it is serious and can result in cardiac failure and death. The syndrome is the result of converting from a catabolic state to an anabolic state. This switch results in profound biochemical changes (e.g. hypophosphataemia, hyponatraemia, hypokalaemia, hypoglycaemia and hypomagnesaemia) that may be fatal in some young people. Clinical features of the refeeding syndrome include delirium, hallucinations, dyspnoea, chest pain, generalised weakness, seizures and coma. Patients are most at risk of the refeeding syndrome in the first week of planned nutrition, and should have daily monitoring of their electrolytes and a daily ECG to assess cardiac risk. This will allow early identification and the introduction of corrections to any biochemical abnormalities.

The outcomes for anorexia nervosa are variable, with the main morbidities being impaired social and psychological functioning (impairing relationships, education and career) and associated mental health difficulties such as depression, anxiety and self-harm. An increased risk of mortality is recognised, and standardised mortality rates of around 3% have been reported. The long-term effects are profound and many of the recorded deaths occur beyond the period of adolescence.

Syllabus Mapping

Adolescent Health/Medicine

- Know about the effects of physical diseases on behaviour and vice versa including somatisation disorders as they occur in secondary care and when to refer to specialist services

- Understand the role of Child and Adolescent Mental Health Services (CAMHS) and know how to refer appropriately

- Be able to assess, diagnose and manage common emotional and behaviour problems such as sleep problems, feeding problems, disruptive behaviour, eating disorders, chronic fatigue syndrome, as they present in secondary care, and understand when to refer to specialist services

References and Further Reading

1. Wood D, Knight C. Anorexia nervosa in adolescents. Paediatrics and Child Health 2015; 25(9): 428–432.

2. Fuentebella J, Kerner JA. Refeeding syndrome. Pediatric Clinics of North America 2009; 56: 1201–1210.

3. Miller HR et al. Anorexia nervosa mortality in Northeast Scotland, 1965–1999. Am J Psychiatry 2005; 162: 753–757.

4. Klein DA, Goldenring JM, Rosen DS, Adelman WP. HEADSSS 3.0: The psychosocial interview for adolescents updated for a new century fuelled by media, Jan 2014. http://contemporarypediatrics.modernmedicine.com/contemporary-pediatrics/content/tags/adolescent-medicine/heeadsss-30-psychosocial-interview

Chapter 8: A disruptive boy
Dr Robert Dinwiddie

A 7 year old boy presents with difficulties at school. He has a very short concentration span and is falling behind in his schoolwork. He is excitable, sometimes disruptive in class, and frequently distracts other children from their work. He does not any have close friends and prefers his own company. His parents say that he is "always on the go" at home.

In the clinic, he is unable to lie still while being examined. He is from a stable family background and there is no past medical or family history of note. There is no evidence of speech or developmental delay.

Physical examination is normal.

Q1. Which of the following is the most likely diagnosis?

Select <u>one</u> answer only

A.   Attention Deficit Hyperactivity Disorder (ADHD)
B.   Autism spectrum disorder
C.   Bipolar disorder
D.   Obsessive-compulsive behaviour
E.   Post-traumatic stress disorder

Q2. If a drug such as methylphenidate were to be used in his treatment, which of the following is the most important side effect?

Select <u>one</u> answer only

A.   Constipation
B.   Decreased appetite and weight loss
C.   Excessive somnolence
D.   Hypotension
E.   Seizures

Answers and Rationale

Q1.   A: Attention Deficit Hyperactivity Disorder (ADHD)
Q2.   B: Decreased appetite and weight loss

This boy has ADHD based on the fact that he is showing the classical core symptoms of hyperactivity, impulsivity and inattention. He is not bipolar because, although he could be described as a "manic" at times, he does not show evidence of depressive phases of behaviour. Autistic spectrum disordered children show a desire to be alone and an "obsession with sameness". His behaviour could also be described as compulsive but not obsessive. Because he is from a stable family and there is no history of domestic, physical or emotional abuse, he does not appear to be suffering from post-traumatic stress disorder.

ADHD is one of the most common psychiatric disorders of childhood and, depending on which diagnostic definition is used, it affects 3–9% of school-age children in the UK (1). It is a heterogeneous behavioural condition characterised by the core symptoms of hyperactivity, impulsivity and inattention. The contribution of each of these features varies from one case to another. In order to make the diagnosis, the behavioural features must be sufficiently severe to cause significant impairment in various settings, including home, school and healthcare facilities (1). ADHD is often seen with other conditions such as alterations of mood, conduct disorders and problems with learning, which may additionally be associated with anxiety disorders and difficulties in communication.

The aetiology is multifactorial. Genetic factors may be important in a significant number of cases. ADHD has an increased frequency in those with neurofibromatosis type 1, Angelman and fragile X syndromes (2, 3). Many cases, however, have features suggestive of an environmental causation related to their socio-economic and family backgrounds. It may also be the case that certain, as yet unrecognised extra-genetic defects can lead to a predisposition to the development of ADHD in vulnerable individuals – the so-called 'epigenetic' effect (4).

Assessment should explore other important causal factors, including extreme poverty, exposure to maternal alcohol and substance abuse in pregnancy, low birthweight and preterm birth. Additional factors could be mental health problems in the parents or family caregivers and exposure to domestic violence or psychological, physical or sexual abuse. A further aspect of the overall assessment should include allowing the child and family to express their own feelings, especially their expectations and involvement in any planned treatment programmes.

Advice should be given on the importance of a nutritionally balanced diet and the value of exercise in general health and wellbeing. If the history suggests certain foods or drinks exacerbate symptoms, then it may be useful to eliminate individual items under the supervision of a dietician. The more general elimination of artificial colourings and additives is not recommended as general treatment for ADHD in this age group (1).

Treatment is based on the severity of symptoms. In mild cases, a period of up to 10 weeks of watchful waiting may be indicated. When it is clear that the symptoms are causing a significant effect on family life, the parents or carers should be offered referral to a parent-training/education programme. This can be commenced either on its own or in conjunction with group cognitive behavioural therapy and/or social skills training for the child (1). Close involvement with the school and local Child and Adolescent Mental Health Services (CAHMS) is vital in all cases, but especially in those with moderate or severe symptoms. Drug treatment is not recommended for preschool children. Children of school age with severe ADHD should be offered drug treatment as first-line therapy, along with a group-based parent training/education programme. Drug treatment should not be used on its own but in association with appropriate psychological, behavioural and educational interventions (1). Methylphenidate is recommended as initial therapy for those with an associated conduct disorder or without comorbidity (1). It is thought to act by increasing dopamine levels in the frontal lobes. The dose should be titrated against tolerability and symptom responsiveness over 4–6 weeks. Significant side effects include appetite suppression and reduced growth velocity. Height and weight should therefore be checked every 6 months. Cardiovascular side effects include tachycardia, arrhythmias and hypertension. Night-time insomnia but not daytime somnolence may occur, as can constipation and tics but not usually seizures. Before commencement of the drug treatment, it is therefore important to carry out a full cardiovascular assessment and documentation of height and weight.

Atomoxetine and dexamfetamine are used for those with other comorbidities or where methylphenidate has been unsuccessful (1). Modified release preparations can be helpful in improving adherence to treatment and avoiding the need for administration at school.

Most patients with long-term symptoms of ADHD will go on to have significant difficulties in adult life. These include personality disorders, difficulties with emotional and social relationships, substance misuse, an increased risk of being unemployed and involvement in criminal activities (2).

Syllabus Mapping

Behavioural medicine/Psychiatry

- Know the signs and symptoms of Attention Deficit Hyperactivity Disorder (ADHD) and the principles of diagnosis and management.

References and Further Reading

1. NICE guidelines (CG72). Attention deficit hyperactivity disorder: Diagnosis and management in children, young people and adults. www.nice.org.uk/cg72.

2. Lewin C. Mental Health. In: Gardiner M, Eisen S, Murphy C (eds). Training in Paediatrics. Oxford University Press: Oxford, 2009: 369–380.

3. Verkuijl N, Perkins M, Fazel M. Childhood attention-deficit/hyperactivity disorder. BMJ 2015; 350: 28–31.

4. Webb E. Poverty, maltreatment and attention deficit hyperactivity disorder. Arch Dis Child 2013; 98: 397–400.

Chapter 9: A tired teenage girl
Dr Robert Dinwiddie

A 14 year old girl is referred due to emotional lability and deteriorating school performance. Her parents say that, over the past few weeks, she has "lost interest" in her normal daily activities. She is irritable with her friends and is making less social contact with them. She previously mixed socially and had a boyfriend, but not now. She had an episode of glandular fever 6 months previously. She appears to lack energy, her appetite is poor and she has given up her regular sports activities. Physical examination is normal and her height and weight are on the 25th centile.

Her puberty is stage 3.

Q1. Which of the following is the most likely diagnosis?

Select <u>one</u> answer only

A.   Anorexia nervosa
B.   Bipolar disorder
C.   Chronic fatigue syndrome/myalgic encephalomyelitis (CFS/ME)
D.   Depression
E.   Early onset schizophrenia

Q2. Which of the following agents has been approved for initial treatment of this condition?

Select <u>one</u> answer only

A.   Fluoxetine
B.   Lithium
C.   Methylphenidate
D.   Olanzapine
E.   Risperidone

Answers and Rationale

Q1.   **D: Depression**
Q2.   **A: Fluoxetine**

This girl is suffering from depression. Although her mood is low, she is not showing signs of hypomania; thus a bipolar disorder can be excluded. Her normal height and weight for her age also make it unlikely that she has anorexia nervosa. There are several reports of depression as a complication of infection with the Epstein-Barr virus. A recent review, however, indicated that it was no more common (5%) than that seen in age-matched controls (1) and it would usually have resolved by this stage in her illness. Depression is also a well-described complication of CFS/ME. A recent study of 542 subjects aged 12–18 years demonstrated a prevalence of 29% (2). This is an unlikely primary diagnosis in her case, because although she is tired, she is not demonstrating other typical features of CFS/ME, such as chronic fatigue and myalgia.

Depression is known to affect 5–6% of young people aged 13–18 (3). It occurs twice as frequently in girls than in boys. An assessment of an affected individual should take into account the social, educational and family background. The patient's interpersonal relationships with their family and friends are particularly important elements in both assessment and treatment. Particular attention should be paid to exposure to any recent undesirable life events, such as bereavement, parental divorce or separation or a severely disappointing personal experience. Other relevant factors may include bullying, physical, emotional or sexual abuse and the misuse of drugs or alcohol. Self-harm can be another major feature, which will require its own particular treatment plan as set out by the National Institute for Health and Care Excellence (NICE) (4). The presence of a history of parental depression increases the risk of a young person developing depression. Treatment in these cases should include involvement of the appropriate adult mental health services for the affected parent.

Those with mild depression can be managed in primary care and the community if appropriately trained professional carers are available. For those with mild depression who do not want intervention and are thought likely to recover, a period of 'watchful waiting' for 2 weeks can be undertaken. Those who are still symptomatic at 4 weeks, without comorbid problems or suicidal ideation, should be offered individual supportive therapy, cognitive behavioural therapy or guided self-help. CAMHS plays a pivotal role in the management of patients with depression, particularly if moderate or severe. It is important that young people being treated for depression build a trusting ongoing relationship with their caregivers, so that they are given age-appropriate information and are involved in treatment decisions. They should also be informed about self-help groups and helplines. Advice regarding general health and wellbeing, particularly in relation to exercise and the need for a healthy diet, are also important.

In the initial NICE guidance (2005) (5), it was recommended that psychological therapies such as individual support therapy, individual or group cognitive behavioural therapy or guided self-help should be used for 2–3 months before the consideration of drug therapy. More recently, NICE (2015) (5, 6) has allowed the use of drug therapy, in conjunction with psychological therapy, as initial treatment in moderate or severe cases. Fluoxetine has been shown to be effective in clinical trials in this age group.

It is a selective serotonin (5 hydroxytryptamine 5-HT) uptake inhibitor (SSRI). Its use may, however, be associated with a small increase in the risk of self-harm and suicidal thoughts, particularly when it is first prescribed. Careful follow-up is therefore required. When used continuously, it has a relatively long half-life of 4–6 days and its active metabolite norfluoxetine of up to 9 days. It is recommended that, when a remission is induced, the drug is continued for 6 months before it is gradually withdrawn (5). Due to its long half-life, active levels will persist for many days after it is stopped.

Lithium is a 'mood-stabilising' drug that is mainly used in the treatment of bipolar disorder. It is less commonly used in the prophylaxis and treatment of *recurrent* unipolar depression. Lithium is also used as concomitant therapy with antidepressant medication in patients who have had an incomplete response to treatment for acute bipolar depression, and to augment other antidepressants in patients with treatment-resistant depression as an unlicensed indication. Drugs such as methylphenidate (and dexamfetamine) are approved for use in the treatment of ADHD but not depression.

Olanzapine can help reduce feelings of anxiety related to issues such as weight and diet in people with anorexia who haven't responded to other treatments, but is not likely to be useful here (as it should have been established that this young person has depression not anorexia). Respiridone is an example of an antipsychotic used in the treatment of schizophrenia but not depression.

Specific longer-term psychological follow-up may be necessary in individual cases where the affected person is at increased risk of relapse or recurrent episodes of depression. Elements relating to this include 2 or more previous episodes, those with high symptom levels in the acute phase of the illness, and exposure to continuing social or family-related increased factors (5).

Syllabus Mapping

Behavioural Medicine/Psychiatry

- Understand the role of Child and Adolescent Mental Health Services (CAHMS) and know how to refer appropriately.

- Be able to assess and diagnose important mental health problems in children and adolescents including depression, psychosis and early onset schizophrenia and understand when to refer to specialist services.

References and Further Reading

1. Malhotra S, Kaur N, Kumar P, Bhatia MS, Hans C. Viral Infections and Depression. Delhi Psychiatry Journal 2012; 15: 188–195.

2. Bould H, Collin S, Lewis G, Rimes K, Crawley E. Depression in paediatric chronic fatigue syndrome. Arch Dis Child 2013; 98: 425–428.

3. Lewin C. Mental Health. In: Gardiner M, Eisen S, Murphy C (eds). Training in Paediatrics. Oxford University Press: Oxford, 2009: 369–380.

4. NICE guidance (CG16). Self-harm. The short-term physical and psychological management and secondary prevention of self-harm in primary and secondary care. www.nice.org.uk/cg16.

5. NICE guidance (CG28). Depression in children and young people: Identification and management in primary, community and secondary care. www.nice.org.uk/cg28.

6. Hopkins K, Crosland P, Elliot N, Bewley S. Diagnosis and management of depression in children and young people: Summary of updated NICE guidance. BMJ 2015; 350: 31–32.

Chapter 10: A blue baby boy
Dr Robert Dinwiddie, Dr Andrew Boon

10

A baby boy, born at term, presents at the age of 6 hours with tachypnoea, persistent cyanosis, lethargy and poor feeding. On examination, his respiratory rate is 60/minute, the chest is clear, and the heart rate is 120/minute. Heart sounds show an ejection systolic murmur at the left upper sternal edge and there is no hepatosplenomegaly.

His oxygen saturation in air is 85%, with no significant increase in 100% oxygen. His chest x-ray shows clear but underperfused lung fields with no cardiomegaly. An ECG shows the normal right ventricular preponderance for his age.

Q1. Which of the following is the most likely diagnosis?

Select <u>one</u> answer only

A.   Coarctation of the aorta
B.   Patent arterial duct
C.   Pulmonary valve stenosis
D.   Tetralogy of Fallot
E.   Ventricular septal defect

Q2. Which of the following treatments will be most effective at this stage?

Select <u>one</u> answer only

A.   Administration of nitric oxide
B.   Infusion of prostaglandin E1
C.   Infusion of tolazoline
D.   Oral captopril
E.   Oral sildenafil

Answers and Rationale

Q1.   C: Pulmonary valve stenosis
Q2.   B: Infusion of prostaglandin E1

The clinical history, physical findings and investigation results in this case suggest that this boy has pulmonary valve stenosis (1). This is further supported by the inability to increase oxygen saturations in 100% inspired oxygen. Coarctation of the aorta and ventricular septal defect would not result in cyanosis at this age. The arterial duct is commonly still patent at this age, but would not result in cyanosis and no murmur would be heard as the pulmonary and systemic pressures are similar on day 1. Tetralogy of Fallot would not present with cyanosis so early in life.

As stated in the history, the chest x-ray will show clear but underperfused lungs. Oxygen saturations show persistent hypoxaemia unresponsive to 100% inspired oxygen. The ECG at this age normally shows relative right ventricular hypertrophy with a frontal QRS axis of around 75º. In the neonatal period, T waves are normally upright in the right ventricular leads V1 or V3R during the first 2 to 3 days of life, but become inverted thereafter. The ECG at this age may therefore not be particularly helpful in establishing the underlying diagnosis, which is most clearly delineated by echocardiography. The main benefit of the ECG is to distinguish between pulmonary atresia with an intact ventricular septum and critical pulmonary valve stenosis. In pulmonary atresia, there is typically evidence of left ventricular hypertrophy (1).

Pulmonary valve stenosis accounts for around 10% of congenital heart disease and it can be valvular, supravalvular or subvalvular in type (1). The pulmonary valve develops during the 7th to 8th week of intrauterine life. The degree of abnormal development at this time is extremely variable, but can result in significant obstruction to the pulmonary outflow tract in the neonatal period (critical/severe pulmonary valve stenosis). After birth, if normal blood flow to the lungs through the pulmonary valve is restricted, it then becomes dependent on a patent arterial duct. As the duct closes, the baby becomes increasingly cyanosed, resulting from the shunting of blood from right to left at atrial level, usually within the first few hours after birth. Two types of critical pulmonary valve stenosis are described – with and without an intact ventricular septum. The incidence of pulmonary valve stenosis with an intact ventricular septum is around 4–6 per 100,000 births. The incidence of pulmonary valve stenosis is increased if there is a family history of similar cardiac lesions and in infants with diabetic mothers.

Initial treatment includes the administration of IV prostaglandin E1. An important side effect of prostaglandin E1 is apnoea. Nitric oxide is a pulmonary vasodilator, so will not help in this situation. Tolazoline and sildenafil reduce pulmonary hypertension, but that is not the primary problem in this case. Similarly, captopril will not be beneficial because it is an afterload reducing agent. Definitive treatment includes balloon valvuloplasty dilation. It has even been performed in utero for cases of pulmonary valve atresia with intact ventricular septum (NICE guidance 2006) (2). In severe cases where valvuloplasty is unsuccessful, a Blalock-Taussig shunt can be performed. In this procedure, a small Gore-Tex tube is placed between the brachiocephalic (innominate) artery and the pulmonary artery, thus mimicking the function of a patent arterial duct. This is usually a temporary procedure until full corrective surgery can take place at a slightly older age.

Congenital cardiac defects occur in 8–10 per 1,000 live births. The approximate incidence of the most common lesions is shown in Table 10.1 (see over).

Table 10.1: Congenital cardiac defect classification and frequency

Acyanotic left-right shunts	Ventricular septal defect (VSD)	20%
	Persistent arterial duct	12%
	Isolated atrial septal defect (ASD)	7%
Obstructive lesions	Pulmonary stenosis (PS)	10%
	Coarctation of aorta (COA)	8%
	Aortic stenosis (AS)	5%
Cyanotic	Tetralogy of Fallot (TOF)	10%
	Transposition of great arteries (TGA)	5%
	Total anomalous pulmonary venous connection (TAPVC)	1%

Adapted from Archer A, Barnes N. Cardiology. In Gardiner M, Eisen S, Murphy C, eds. Teaching in Paediatrics. Oxford University Press: Oxford, 2009: 73-92, with permission.

Syllabus Mapping

Neonatology

- Be able to assess, diagnose and manage congenital anomalies presenting in the neonatal period and make appropriate referrals.

Cardiology

- Know the various presentations of congenital heart problems at all ages and be able to assess, diagnose and manage and make appropriate referrals.

References and Further Reading

1. Archer A, Barnes N. Cardiology. In: Gardiner M, Eisen S, Murphy C (eds). Training in Paediatrics. Oxford University Press: Oxford, 2009: 73–92.

2. Percutaneous fetal balloon valvuloplasty for pulmonary atresia with intact ventricular septum. NICE interventional procedure guidance [IPG176] May 2006.

Chapter 11: A 2 year old with severe stridor
Dr Judith Gilchrist

A 2 year old boy presents to the emergency department with breathing difficulties. His mother says the child was well when dropped off at nursery that morning but when she collected him later that day, she noticed some noisy breathing that had worsened over the course of several hours. The child has no significant past medical history and no previous episodes of croup. There was no history of witnessed choking. He was fully immunised.

Initial triage observations show a temperature of 37.1°C, a heart rate of 150/minute, a respiratory rate of 52/minute, with a central capillary refill time 2 seconds and oxygen saturation 90% in air. On examination, he is agitated with stridor, marked recession and tracheal tug, no wheeze, symmetrical chest movement and poor air entry bilaterally.

Q1. What would be the first three steps in management?

Select three answers only

A.   Arrange urgent portable chest x-ray
B.   Arrange an x-ray of the lateral soft tissue neck
C.   Call for anaesthetic help
D.   Give high-flow oxygen via a non-rebreather mask
E.   Give IM adrenaline
F.   Give nebulised adrenaline
G.   Give nebulised budesonide
H.   Give oral dexamethasone
I.   Site IV cannula and give cefotaxime
J.   Site IV cannula and give hydrocortisone

Q2. What is the most likely cause of this child's respiratory distress?

Select one answer only

A.   Bacterial tracheitis
B.   Epiglottitis
C.   Foreign body
D.   Retropharyngeal abscess
E.   Viral croup

Answers and Rationale

Q1. **C: Call for anaesthetic help**
D: Give high-flow oxygen via non-rebreather mask
F: Give nebulised adrenaline
Q2. **C: Foreign body**

This child is presenting with severe stridor, representing upper airway compromise and threatened upper airway obstruction. He is hypoxic with falling saturations and agitation. Whatever the underlying cause, the initial emergency management would be the same – which is giving oxygen, buying time with nebulised adrenaline, and calling for senior anaesthetic and probably ENT help. Other definitive treatments would depend on the cause. It is useful to consider the inappropriate options in this case.

Stridor is a sign of upper airway obstruction. Generally, inspiratory stridor suggests laryngeal obstruction whereas expiratory stridor suggests obstruction in the lower trachea. Biphasic stridor suggests a glottic or subglottic problem with less flexibility in the airway wall.

A. A chest x-ray is unlikely to be helpful as the pathology described is most likely to be in the upper airway.

B. A lateral x-ray of the neck might be helpful in making a diagnosis of retropharyngeal abscess or might suggest acute epiglottitis. However, there is a significant risk of disturbing the child and precipitating acute upper airway obstruction during an x-ray.

E. IM adrenaline would be appropriate for an anaphylactic cause, but there is nothing in the history or examination to suggest this – a shorter history would be likely, a past history of allergies might be expected, and some other features of anaphylaxis, especially swelling and circulatory effects, would generally be seen.

G and H. Nebulised budesonide or oral dexamethasone are both appropriate treatments for a mild-to-moderate viral croup, but, in this case, the priority is to secure the airway. These treatments will take at least 90 minutes to begin to take effect.

I and J. Siting an IV cannula for any purpose should be deferred until the airway is secure or at least until a senior anaesthetist is present, as it again risks precipitating complete obstruction.

There are a number of possible causes of acute stridor.

Croup

This is a viral upper respiratory infection causing inflammation around the vocal cords. Typically, the child is not particularly unwell, has a mild fever, with the onset or a worsening often late in the evening after the child has gone to bed. Although it usually causes mild symptoms of a barking cough and mild stridor, it can rarely cause severe airway narrowing. Because it is, by far, the most common cause of stridor, it thus becomes one of the most common causes of severe airway compromise. Specific treatment in addition to the emergency measures above is steroids – usually oral dexamethasone or nebulised budesonide, which are of equal efficacy, and probably more effective than prednisolone (1, 2).

Bacterial tracheitis

As its name suggests this is a bacterial infection of the trachea and larynx, the most common organisms being *Staphylococcus aureus* and *Streptococcus pyogenes*, but many other organisms have been described as causative. These children present as looking toxic with high fevers and often with a prodrome of a mild upper respiratory infection. They will often progress rapidly and require intubation to secure the airway as well as supportive intensive care with broad-spectrum antibiotics (3).

Epiglottitis

This has a very similar presentation to bacterial tracheitis, but is now rarely seen since the introduction of the Hib vaccine. There is usually no prodrome, but a rapid onset of severe symptoms. The classic presentation is a triad of dysphagia, drooling and physical distress, and biphasic stridor may be seen. The management is the same as bacterial tracheitis.

Foreign body

While there is often a history of choking to suggest a foreign body causing stridor, absence of a clear history doesn't rule it out. In the real case on which this question is based, this was indeed the cause. The child had, unwitnessed, swallowed a paperclip that had become lodged at the vocal cords, causing oedema that worsened over several hours. Oxygen and nebulised adrenaline bought time for the anaesthetist to prepare for intubation and, following gaseous induction, the lodged paper clip was removed by Magill's forceps.

A foreign body near the upper airway is most likely to present acutely, but can present some days or weeks after the event if it becomes lodged in the soft tissue and leads to an abscess formation.

Rarer causes of stridor

Other rare causes of acute stridor that should be considered include anaphylaxis, diphtheria, hypocalcaemia, trauma (laryngeal fracture), retropharyngeal abscess and TB. A retropharyngeal abscess is the most common in children under 5. It can present with a sore throat, fever, neck stiffness and stridor. An abscess develops following direct or lymphatic spread of upper respiratory or oral infections. Diphtheria is very rare in Europe due to the successful immunisation programme. It is caused by *Corynebacterium diphtheriae*. It primarily infects the upper respiratory tract and causes upper airway obstruction via toxin-mediated production of a pseudomembrane across the upper airway.

Blunt laryngeal trauma is much rarer in children than in adults. There will usually be a history of trauma to the anterior neck and signs ranging from mild dysphonia to severe stridor and respiratory distress. Signs could include anterior neck bruising, loss of laryngeal landmarks, oedema, surgical emphysema or palpable cartilage fractures. Protection of the unstable airway is paramount in management.

Hypocalcaemia can cause a laryngospasm rather than true stridor, due to tetany of the vocal cords. This has been reported in neonates secondary to maternal vitamin D deficiency (4). A rare cause in older children may be hypocalcaemia secondary to autoimmune hypoparathyroidism.

Syllabus Mapping

Emergency medicine including Accidents and Poisoning

- Be able to assess, diagnose and manage children presenting with anaphylaxis including acute life-threatening upper airways obstruction

Respiratory Medicine with ENT

- Be able to assess, diagnose and manage stridor

References and Further Reading

1. Geelhoed G, Macdonald W. Oral and inhaled steroids in croup: A randomised, placebo-controlled trial. Pediatr Pulmonol 1995; 20: 355–61.

2. Sparrow A, Geelhoed G. Prednisolone vs dexamethasone in the treatment of croup: A randomised equivalence trial. J Paediatr Child Health 2003; 39(6): A8.

3. Al-Mutairi B, Kirk V. Bacterial tracheitis in children: Approach to diagnosis and treatment. Paediatr Child Health 2004; 9: 25–30.

4. D Sharma, A Pandita, OT Pratap, S Murki. Laryngospasm and neonatal seizure due to hypocalcaemia and vitamin D deficiency. BMJ Case Reports 2014. doi: bcr-2014-206795.

Chapter 12: A 3 month old girl with diarrhoea
Dr Robert Dinwiddie, Dr Helyeh Sadreddini

(12)

A 3 month old girl presents with a history of irritability, vomiting and recurrent, occasionally blood-stained, loose stools. She was born at term, with a birthweight of 3.5 kg. She has been largely breastfed with occasional top-up formula feeds.

On examination, she is clinically well but irritable on handling. Her weight is 4.9 kg (9th centile). She has small patches of eczema on her arms and legs. Her abdomen is soft, but perineal redness is noted.

Q1. Which of the following is the most likely diagnosis?

Select <u>one</u> answer only

A.   Congenital lactase deficiency
B.   Cow's milk protein allergy
C.   Eosinophilic oesophagitis
D.   Gastro-oesophageal reflux
E.   Meckel's diverticulum

Q2. Which of the following milk formulas is initially most appropriate in this case?

Select <u>one</u> answer only

A.   Amino acid based
B.   Extensively hydrolysed cow's milk
C.   Goat's milk based
D.   Lactose free
E.   Soya based

Answers and Rationale

Q1.   **B: Cow's milk protein allergy**
Q2.   **B: Extensively hydrolysed cow's milk**

Cow's milk protein allergy is the most likely diagnosis in this case (1, 2). The symptoms of cow's milk protein allergy vary, and can include food refusal, vomiting, food impaction in the oesophagus and poor growth. Loose bloody stools are a recognised feature. Of the other options available: Congenital lactase deficiency would present from birth with diarrhoea because such infants are unable to digest the lactose in breast milk (2). Eosinophilic oesophagitis might mimic some of the symptoms but this recently recognised allergic/autoimmune condition that can occur at any age is relatively rare in all age groups (see below for a further brief discussion). Gastro-oesophageal reflux could result in recurrent vomiting and irritability, but is less likely to result in loose, occasionally blood-stained, stools. Meckel's diverticulum could cause blood-stained stools but not vomiting and irritability.

Cow's milk protein allergy is the most common food allergy in the paediatric age group, affecting up to 7.5% of children. Even when we restrict studies of incidences to those where milk allergy has been proven by food challenge, the incidence is 1% among UK children (3). Most children present before 6 months of age and it rarely presents after 1 year of age, although this does happen. It is hugely variable in its presentation, with some infants or children developing anaphylaxis after exposure to very small amounts while others only develop symptoms after ingestion of much larger amounts of 100–200 ml.

Two distinct types are recognised: IgE- and non-IgE-mediated reactions and when allergy is confirmed by food challenge, non-IgE-mediated reactions are slightly more common in UK children. IgE-mediated (type 1 – immediate hypersensitivity) reactions are typically quick to manifest following exposure, and symptoms develop acutely usually within minutes to 2 hours of drinking the milk or eating foods containing cow's milk protein. Often the feeding history is very helpful, as symptoms frequently coincide with the withdrawal of exclusive breastfeeding or at the introduction of solids (1, 2).

IgE-mediated reactions are most common in atopic individuals, especially those who have a family history of food allergy. Symptoms include swelling of the lips, tongue and periorbital region, itching of the tongue and eyes with conjunctival redness, sneezing, coughing and rhinorrhoea. In this scenario, it should be remembered that the symptoms described can occur even in the absence of a specific allergic trigger. In severe cases, anaphylaxis can develop with acute, sometimes life-threatening, symptoms such as an upper airway obstruction, wheeze, dyspnoea, nausea, vomiting, pallor and collapse.

If allergy to a specific allergen is suspected, then this can be tested for using skin prick testing initially. If this is inconclusive, then further testing such as measurement of total and specific IgE to cow's milk protein and then an oral cow's milk challenge could be conducted. Skin prick tests utilise an extract of the specific allergen and are compared to a positive (histamine) and a negative (saline) control. A wheal diameter of 3 mm or more indicates a positive result. Cow's milk specific IgE levels of >15 kUA/l in 5 year old children have a 95% predictive value (4, 5). Treatment involves avoidance of exposure to cow's milk in the diet, prescription of an oral antihistamine for use in acute events and, in those with severe reactions, an adrenaline auto-injector.

The second type of reaction in infants, such as in this case, is one of non-IgE-mediated cow's milk protein allergy. This has had various names in the literature and some authors had previously labelled this condition as cow's milk protein intolerance. Symptoms usually begin within 4 weeks of starting formula feeds and may not be seen for several hours after the ingestion of cow's milk protein. The most common presenting features are vomiting, colic, mucousy blood-stained stools, faltering growth and anaemia. Proctocolitis is another presenting feature.

These symptoms are also well described in cases of purely breastfed infants, as breast milk does contain small amounts of intact cow's milk protein. The precise incidence is unknown but it may affect up to 1 in 200 breast fed babies in the UK. Management consists of the avoidance of cow's milk protein in the diet, including the mother if she is still breastfeeding, and the substitution of an extensively hydrolysed cow's milk formula (eHF) or (in severe cases) an amino acid based formula. A lactose-free formula is not indicated, as it will not deal with the primary problem. Goat's milk and soya-based formulas are also contraindicated due to a significant incidence of cross-reactive allergy in cow's milk allergic individuals (6).

Most infants and children outgrow their allergy to cow's milk by the age of 18 months to 5 years, but a significant proportion go on to develop other atopic illnesses including hay fever and asthma.

Rarer causes of similar presentations

Eosinophilic oesophagitis is a rare condition, but one that is increasingly recognised in clinical practice (7). The symptoms are often rather non-specific, particularly in younger children. It can present with faltering growth, food refusal, vomiting and apparent pain or discomfort on swallowing. The diagnosis can be confirmed endoscopically, with the histopathology revealing an eosinophilic infiltration of the oesophagus. Treatment depends on the associated pathologies but includes the elimination of known dietary triggers (patient-specific) and steroids (oral budesonide).

A further condition, which is quite rare but again difficult to diagnose, is Food protein-induced enterocolitis syndrome (FPIES). This is most common in children under 9 months of age but does not occur in exclusively breastfed children. In these cases, symptoms present within 2 hours of a feed and include vomiting, lethargy and diarrhoea, which are sometimes severe enough to cause life-threatening shock from gastrointestinal fluid loss secondary to inflammation. The diagnosis of FPIES can be a challenge, as IgE testing and skin prick tests are usually negative. Diagnosis is usually made based on medical history and examination. A low albumin and high neutrophil and platelet counts can be present and a supervised food challenge may need to be considered.

Syllabus Mapping

Gastroenterology

- Be able to assess, diagnose and manage chronic diarrhoea and its complications

Infection, Immunity and Allergy

- Be able to assess, diagnose and manage allergies

References and Further Reading

1. Klein N, Neth O, Eisen S. Infection and immunity. In: Gardiner M, Eisen S, Murphy C (eds). Training in Paediatrics. Oxford University Press: Oxford, 2009: 307-44.

2. Burridge R, Nanduri V. In: Royal College of Paediatrics and Child Health. Clinical Cases for MRCPCH Theory and Science. London, 2014; ch45: 177-179.

3. Schoemaker AA et al. Incidence and natural history of challenge-proven cow's milk protein allergy in European children: EuroPrevall birth cohort study. Allergy 2015; 70: 963-972.

4. Steele C, Conlon N, Edgar JD. Diagnosis of immediate food allergy. BMJ 2014; 349: 32-33.

5. Koletzco S et al. Diagnostic approach and management of cow's milk protein allergy in infants and children: ESPGHAN GI Committee Practical Guidelines. JPGN 2012; 55: 221-229.

6. Liacouras C et al. Eosinophilic esophagitis: Updated consensus, recommendations for children and adults. JACI 2011; 3-20.

7. Luyt D, Ball H, Makwana N, Green MR, Bravin K, Nasser SM, Clark AT. BSACI guideline for the diagnosis and management of cows' milk allergy. Clin Exp Allergy 2014: 44; 642-672.

Chapter 13: A 6 month old boy with fits
Dr Poothirikovil Venugopalan

(13)

A previously well 6 month old boy presents with generalised fits intermittently for the last 1 hour. He received buccal midazolam twice in the ambulance without relief. On arrival in hospital, he has intravenous lorazepam, which controlled his fits. There is no history of preceding fever, and his development is normal. There is no family history of epilepsy. He is admitted to the ward where his observations show a temperature 37°C, heart rate 140/minute, respiratory rate 30/minute, capillary refill time 2 seconds, oxygen saturation 95% in air, and blood pressure 80/50 mmHg. His blood investigations show:

Haemoglobin	115 g/l
White cell count	10 x 10⁹/l
Platelets	400 x 10⁹/l
CRP	4 mg/l
Sodium	139 mmol/l
Potassium	5.2 mmol/l
Urea	3.3 mmol/l
Creatinine	30 µmol/l
Calcium	1.2 mmol/l
Magnesium	0.8 mmol/l (0.6–1)
Phosphate	1.2 mmol/l (1.3–2.6)
Albumin	35 mg/l (0–40)
Bilirubin – total	17 umol/l
ALT	30 U/l
AST	50 U/l (8–60)
ALP	1200 U/l (59–425)

Q1. Which of the following is the most likely diagnosis?

Select <u>one</u> answer only

A.   Hypoparathyroidism
B.   Intestinal malabsorption
C.   Liver disease
D.   Nutritional rickets
E.   Renal failure

The fits recur as soon as he is transferred to the ward.

Q2. What would be your first line of management?

Select <u>one</u> answer only

A.   Buccal midazolam
B.   IV calcium gluconate
C.   IV lorazepam
D.   IV phenytoin
E.   Rectal diazepam

Answers and Rationale

Q1.   D: Nutritional rickets
Q2.   B: IV calcium gluconate

This is a previously well, 6 month old boy, who presents with prolonged fits that are controlled with intravenous lorazepam. He has stable observations. From the clinical presentation, the 2 common possibilities would be febrile fits and the first presentation of epilepsy. However, his temperature was normal, and he was well prior to the onset of the fits. Moreover, the blood results show a less common cause for the fits.

The blood results are shown here with the normal values in brackets.

Haemoglobin	115 g/l (110–140)
White cell count	10 x 10⁹/l (6–15)
Platelets	400 x 10⁹/l (150–450)
CRP	4 mg/l (<10)
Sodium	139 mmol/l (133–146)
Potassium	5.2 mmol/l (3.5–5.5)
Urea	3.3 mmol/l (0.8–5.5)
Creatinine	30 µmol/l (13–39)
Calcium	1.2 mmol/l (2.2–2.7)
Magnesium	0.8 mmol/l (0.6–1)
Phosphate	1.2 mmol/l (1.3–2)
Albumin	35 mg/l (30–45)
Bilirubin – total	17 umol/l (0–21)
ALT	30 U/l (0–41)
AST	50 U/l (8–60)
ALP	1200 U/l (59–425)

These results show low serum calcium, slightly low phosphate, and elevated alkaline phosphatase, features that are consistent with rickets. A blood gas analysis would show low ionised calcium, which triggered the fits. Seizures are being increasingly recognised as a presenting feature of nutritional rickets (1). Once you attend to the airway, breathing and circulation, the first line of treatment would be intravenous calcium gluconate, as low serum calcium is the most likely cause of the fits. While infusing calcium, it is important to make sure the intravenous access is well functioning, as extravasation of calcium into the soft tissues can lead to tissue damage. However, if there is delay in getting or administering calcium, the fits can be stopped with an anticonvulsant as a temporary measure. Such a measure may be required even if treatment with intravenous calcium gluconate has been commenced, as it takes time to correct the serum calcium level in the body. However, anticonvulsant therapy is indicated only if the fits are prolonged, generally more than 5 minutes. Intravenous lorazepam would then be the first choice, provided that intravenous access is already established.

It is important to follow the local guidelines or the advanced paediatric life support (APLS) guidelines for the management of seizures. Senior paediatric help should be sought at an early stage. If fits persist, or there is difficulty in normalising serum calcium, consultation with a tertiary specialist is recommended.

Nutritional rickets

The primary cause of rickets is vitamin D deficiency. Vitamin D is required for calcium absorption from the gut. Vitamin D stores arise from 2 sources: sunlight and diet. The ultraviolet rays in the sunlight convert a precursor of vitamin D (5-dihydrotachysterol) present in the skin to vitamin D (cholecalciferol). The vitamin D produced or absorbed from the gut is converted to 25-hydroxycholecalciferol in the liver and further to 1,25-dihydrocholecalciferol in the kidneys, which is the biologically active form of the vitamin. Dietary sources include butter, eggs, fish liver oils, margarine, fortified milk and juice, mushrooms, and oily fish such as tuna, herring, and salmon. All infant milk formulas and dairy products are fortified with vitamin D and form an important source (2).

Vitamin D deficiency can result from insufficient production in the body due to the sun's ultraviolet light not reaching the skin. This can occur due to the use of strong sunblock, too much 'covering up' in the sunlight, or not getting out into the sun. People with darker skins may need more sunlight to maintain vitamin D levels. In some ethnic groups, mothers avoid exposure to the sun for religious or cultural reasons, leading to a maternal shortage of vitamin D. Human milk contains little vitamin D, generally less than 20–40 IU/l. Therefore, infants who are breastfed are at risk for rickets. Furthermore, maternal deficiency results in low vitamin D stores in the newborn, as well as also a further reduction in vitamin D in breast milk (3-5).

Vitamin D is essential for absorption of calcium from the gut, and deficiency leads to hypocalcaemia, which stimulates excess secretion of the parathyroid hormone. In turn, renal phosphorus loss is enhanced, further reducing the deposition of calcium in bones. Hypocalcaemia manifests itself as a central nervous system irritability and poor muscular contractility. Low calcium levels decrease the threshold of excitation of neurons, leading to neuronal excitability (sensory and motor), paraesthesias, tetany (i.e. contractions of the muscles of the hands, arms, feet, larynx, bronchioles), seizures, and even psychiatric changes in children. Cardiac function may also be impaired due to poor muscle contractility, including prolongation of the QTc interval (1).

Excess parathyroid hormone also produces changes in the bone similar to those occurring in hyperparathyroidism. Early in the course of rickets, the calcium concentration in the serum decreases. After the parathyroid response, the calcium concentration usually returns to normal, though phosphorus levels remain low. Alkaline phosphatase, which is produced by overactive osteoblast cells, leaks into the extracellular fluids, so that its concentration rises to anywhere from moderate elevation to very high levels.

Table 13.1: Causes of hypocalcaemia in infancy

Pathophysiology	Causes
Hypoparathyroidism	• Aplasia or hypoplasia of parathyroid gland • Di George (22q11 deletion) syndrome • Fetal exposure to retinoic acid • VACTERL complex (vertebral defects, anal atresia, tracheoesophageal fistula with (o)esophageal atresia, and renal and limb abnormalities) • CHARGE association (coloboma, heart defects, choanal atresia, renal abnormalities, growth retardation, male genital anomalies, and ear abnormalities) • Parathyroid hormone (PTH) receptor defects Pseudohypoparathyroidism • Autoimmune parathyroiditis • Infiltrations – Haemosiderosis, Wilson disease, thalassaemia
Vitamin D abnormalities	• Vitamin D deficiency – Dietary insufficiency and maternal use of anticonvulsants • Acquired or inherited disorders of the vitamin D metabolism • Resistance to actions of vitamin D • Liver disease – Liver disease can affect 25-hydroxylation of vitamin D; certain drugs (e.g. phenytoin, carbamazepine, phenobarbital, isoniazid, and rifampin) can increase the activity of P-450 enzymes, which can increase the 25-hydroxylation as well as the catabolism of vitamin D
Hyperphosphataemia	• Excessive phosphate intake from feeding of cow's milk or infant formula with improper (low) calcium to phosphate ratio • Excessive phosphate or inappropriate calcium to phosphate ratio in total parenteral nutrition • Renal failure

Other causes	• Malabsorption syndromes
	• Alkalosis – Respiratory alkalosis is caused by hyperventilation; metabolic alkalosis occurs with the administration of bicarbonate, diuretics, or chelating agents, such as the high doses of citrates taken in during massive blood transfusions
	• Pancreatitis
	• Hungry bones syndrome – Rapid skeletal mineral deposition is seen in infants with rickets or hypoparathyroidism after starting vitamin D therapy

Other causes of rickets

Intestinal malabsorption, as in coeliac disease and diseases of the liver or kidney, may produce the clinical and secondary biochemical picture of nutritional rickets. Anticonvulsant drugs (e.g. phenobarbital, phenytoin) accelerate the metabolism of vitamin D, which may lead to insufficiency and rickets.

This child has normal haemoglobin and serum albumin levels, which exclude coeliac disease as a cause. Renal function ALT and AST are normal, excluding the possibility of liver or renal disease as a cause of rickets and hypocalcaemia.

A rare X-linked dominant form exists called vitamin D-resistant rickets or X-linked hypophosphataemia, where there is excessive renal loss of phosphate, leading to a state of vitamin D resistance. Generally, the liver enzymes are normal in these children and the serum phosphate levels very low. Another noteworthy feature of this condition is the near normal serum calcium level.

Syllabus mapping

Nutrition

- Be able to assess, diagnose and manage specific vitamin and micronutrient deficiencies

References and Further Reading

1. Gad K, Khan M, Mahmood K. Afebrile seizures and electrocardiography abnormality: An unusual presentation of nutritional rickets. Scott Med J 2014; 59: e16–e19.

2. Shaw DN. Prevention and treatment of nutritional rickets. J Steroid Biochem Mol Biol 2015; 19.pii: S0960-0760(15)30116-3. doi: 10.1016/j.jsbmb.2015.10.014

3. Allgrove J, Mughal MZ. Calcium deficiency rickets: extending the spectrum of 'nutritional' rickets. Arch Dis Child 2014; 99: 794–5.

4. Thacher TD, Fischer PR, Tebben PJ et al. Increasing incidence of nutritional rickets: A population-based study in Olmsted County, Minnesota. Mayo Clin Proc 2013; 88: 176–83

Chapter 14: A 6 year old boy presenting with pallor
Dr Andrew Maxted, Dr Andrew Lunn

(14)

A 6 year old boy is admitted with pallor and tiredness and ongoing diarrhoea. He was sleeping more than usual and his appetite and drinking had diminished. His urinary output had slowed. He had been unwell a week earlier with a 3 day episode of abdominal pain, diarrhoea and vomiting, but the bloody diarrhoea, although still present, was improving. He had previously been well. On examination, he is pale and quiet. There is no evidence of a rash or other cutaneous lesions. His temperature is 38.3°C and his heart rate is 140/minute. His blood pressure is 120/75 mmHg. Heart sounds are normal. The respiratory examination is normal. An examination of the abdomen shows a mild degree of generalised tenderness and a 2 cm palpable liver. Blood tests show:

Haemoglobin	79 g/l
MCV	72 fl
MCH	27 pg (23–31)
MCHC	320 g/dl (32–35)
White cell count	14.2 x 10^9/l
Platelets	19 x 10^9/l
Clotting	normal
Sodium	148 mmol/l
Potassium	6.5 mmol/l
Urea	24.8 mmol/l
Creatinine	240 μmol/l
Glucose	7.2 mmol/l
Calcium	2.5 mmol/l
Phosphate	1.9 mmol/l
ALT	37 U/l (0–29)
AST	59 U/l (8–60)
Bilirubin	42 μmol/l
Albumin	36 g/l

Q1. Which is the likely causative agent for this clinical presentation?

Select one answer only

A.   Campylobacter coli
B.   Clostridium difficile
C.   E. coli
D.   Salmonella enterica
E.   Yersinia enterocolitica

Q2. Which of the following is a recognised complication?

Select one answer only

A.   Pancreatitis
B.   Pelvic abscess
C.   Septic arthritis
D.   Subphrenic abscess
E.   Ulcerative colitis

Answers and Rationale

Q1.   **C: E. coli**
Q2.   **A: Pancreatitis**

The clinical story suggests an inflammatory or infective process. The laboratory result indicates a haemolytic anaemia with a low haemoglobin and a raised bilirubin as well as thrombocytopaenia. The clinical chemistry results show acute kidney injury. This would be consistent with a diagnosis of haemolytic-uraemic syndrome (HUS) (1, 2). The most likely organism would be the Shiga-toxin-producing *E. coli* (STEC) O157 (3).

The underlying pathological process is that of a microangiopathy leading to ischaemia. This can cause systemic involvement, including pancreatitis, encephalopathy and myocarditis. It is not associated with a purulent bacterial infection. Ulcerative colitis is a different pathological process altogether.

Haemolytic uraemic syndrome

HUS consists of a triad of microangiopathic haemolytic anaemia, thrombocytopaenia and acute kidney injury. Over 95% of children have a preceding diarrhoeal illness and 83% have been associated with STEC O157. Around 800–900 children in the UK develop a STEC O157 infection each year and, of these, 10–15% go on to develop HUS.

The main vectors for STEC are cows (through infection via undercooked ground meat and unpasteurised fresh milk) and visits to contaminated environments such as farms.Worldwide, *Shigella dysenteriae* is also an important cause of STEC-associated HUS.

HUS should be considered in any child presenting with bloody diarrhoea, and both HUS and infectious causes of bloody diarrhoea are notifiable diseases. The local public health authority should be notified as soon as possible after a potential diagnosis is raised. HUS rarely occurs without diarrhoea, and alternative explanations such complement abnormalities should be sought.

HUS is a disease of microvasculature and predominantly affects the kidneys, with acute kidney injury being identified in the majority of cases. Vascular injury from the endotoxins combine with genetic predispositions to cause endothelial damage. This damage leads to microvascular thrombosis and platelet consumption. Within this, red blood cells are damaged, causing fragmented red blood cells (producing schistocytes on a blood film). Ultimately, this process causes microangiopathic haemolytic anaemia, thrombocytopaenia and glomerular injury, leading to acute kidney injury.

Typically, there is a prodrome of bloody diarrhoea and usually vomiting that can occur 3–14 days after exposure to infection. It is therefore important to obtain a detailed history that covers the previous 2 weeks and that specifically asks about exposure to possible sources of infection.

Haemolytic anaemia and thrombocytopaenia precede the development of acute kidney injury and thus, at an early stage in the disease process, the child may still have near normal urine output but be clinically dehydrated due to the presence of ongoing diarrhoea and vomiting (4). Rarely, children may present with acute hypovolaemic shock. As the disease progresses, the child may develop oliguria or anuria with serum biochemical evidence of acute kidney injury. Consequently, they can become oedematous or overhydrated and their fluid status should be reviewed regularly.

Due to the anaemia and acute disease process, the child will present with pallor, lethargy and occasionally jaundice. Extra-renal manifestations may develop, and around 20% of children can have central nervous system involvement with seizures, reduced consciousness levels and coma (5). Involvement of the GI tract may produce haemorrhagic colitis, pancreatitis and rectal prolapse. Angiopathy, including the small vessels of the heart, will lead to cardiac dysfunction.

All children presenting with bloody diarrhoea of unknown aetiology require a full blood count and film, electrolytes, urea, liver function tests, clotting screen, urinalysis and urgent stool culture. Serum samples must also be sent for E. coli serology and clotted, and EDTA samples stored for further analysis before any transfusions are given (6). Clinical suspicion should remain until 14 days after the diarrhoeal illness. The main focus of management of the patient with HUS is supportive, as there are no specific treatments available for STEC-associated disease. Judicious fluid management is important to avoid under- or over-hydration and it is also important to avoid antibiotics, NSAIDs and anti-motility agents before a diagnosis is confirmed (7). All children will require the input and advice of a paediatric nephrologist, and most will require transfer to a tertiary centre when appropriate and safe to do so.

Transfused platelets are quickly consumed and should be avoided unless there is an acute clinical need, such as a need for surgery or a spontaneous intracranial bleed. Blood transfusions should only be given for symptomatic anaemia. Prevention is also a key part of management and early involvement of the Health Protection Agency allows contact and source tracing. Safe food handling and careful hand washing can also prevent the progression of the disease among the local population.

Mortality for STEC-associated HUS is under 2%, and a recent survey showed renal recovery in 88% of diarrhoea-associated HUS. Poor prognostic indicators include younger children, high neutrophilia at presentation, initial shock and HUS not associated with STEC-producing organisms (where renal recovery is 56%).

Syllabus Mapping

Nephro-urology

- Be able to assess, diagnose and manage nephro-urological disorders, including those with systemic manifestations and make appropriate referral

- Be able to assess, diagnose and manage acute and chronic renal failure

References and Further Reading

1. Noris M, Remuzzi G. Hemolytic Uremic Syndrome. J Am Soc Nephrol 2005; 16: 1035–1050.

2. Lynn RM et al. Childhood Hemolytic Uremic Syndrome: United Kingdom and Ireland. Emergency Infectious Diseases 2005; 11:590-596.

3. Fitzpatrick M. Haemolytic uraemic syndrome and E coli 0157. The management of acute bloody diarrhoea potentially caused by vero cytotoxin-producing Escherichia coli in children. BMJ 1999; 318: 684–5.

4. Trachtman H. HUS and TTP in children. Pediatric Clinics of North America 2013; 60: 1513–1526.

5. Kwon N et al. Acute neurological involvement in diarrhea-associated hemolytic uremic syndrome. Clin J Am Soc Nephrol 2010; 5:1218.

6. Rees L et al. Paediatric nephrology, 2nd edition. Oxford University Press, 2012.

7. https://www.gov.uk/government/uploads/system/uploads/attachment_data/file/342344/management_of_acute_bloody_diarrhoea.pdf.

Chapter 15: A 10 year old boy with tiredness and lethargy
Dr Poothirikovil Venugopalan

(15)

A 10 year old boy, who had been previously well, presents with tiredness and lethargy for the last 6 months. Clinical examination shows no pallor, clubbing or lymphadenopathy, and systemic examination is unremarkable. He weighs 70 kg, and has a height of 140 cm (BMI 35 kg /m²).

15.1: Growth Chart

Q1. Which of the following is the most likely diagnosis?

Select <u>one</u> answer only

A.   Diabetes mellitus
B.   Hypothyroidism
C.   Intracranial space-occupying lesion
D.   Nutritional obesity
E.   Pubertal growth spurt

Q2. What is the most important investigation at this stage?

Select <u>one</u> answer only

A.   MRI brain scan
B.   Echocardiogram
C.   Glycosylated haemoglobin (HbA₁c)
D.   Lipid profile
E.   Thyroid function test

Answers and Rationale

Q1. **D: Nutritional obesity**
Q2. **C: Glycosylated haemoglobin HbA_1c**

The striking abnormality here is the presence of general symptomatology with a high BMI (>25 kg/m² is overweight and >30 kg/m² is obesity), and the absence of any physical findings that would point to an underlying organic pathology as the cause. The growth chart shows that he was on the 50th centile for height and weight from birth to 7 years, and then progressively crossed the centiles upwards to come to above the 99.9th centile in both height and weight. The weight is more affected than the height, and the BMI is in the 'obesity' range. Lethargy and tiredness can be the result of overweight/obesity, and these can also make the condition worse by reduced activity and excessive food intake.

Although tiredness can be an early symptom of type 2 diabetes mellitus, the information available does not suggest a diagnosis of diabetes mellitus, and hence is not the right answer. Hypothyroidism causes weight gain, but the height remains unaffected and hence will not fit this situation. Intracranial space-occupying lesions generally cause an increase in weight, but this boy is systemically well and does not exhibit any abnormal neurology, although the weight gain has been going on for 3 years. Pubertal growth spurt can be a differential diagnosis, but, in this boy, the changes in growth rate have started at the age of 7 years, too early for a puberty-related growth spurt. Moreover, a detailed physical examination to look for pubertal status and for excess fat would make the diagnosis clear.

In view of the tiredness and obesity, this child would benefit from investigations to assess his glucose metabolism, including urine for glucose, fasting blood glucose and HbA_1c, and a detailed analysis of his diet and physical activity profile. A blood pressure record is also essential. In view of the normal neurological examination, a brain scan would not help at this stage. Similarly, an echocardiogram is not indicated. Lipid profile and thyroid function tests are definitely indicated and can be performed on the same blood sample, but would not rank as the most important test.

Nutritional obesity is a common disorder in children. In 2013, WHO estimated that 42 million children under the age of 5 were overweight or obese (1). In the UK, over 30% of children aged 2 to 15 years were overweight or obese (2). Once considered a high-income country problem, overweight and obesity are now on the rise in low- and middle-income countries, particularly in urban settings. In developing countries with emerging economies (classified by the World Bank as lower- and middle-income countries), the rate of increase of childhood overweight and obesity has been more than 30% higher than that of developed countries. The complications are summarised in Table 15.2 (overleaf).

Obesity and overweight are the result of an energy imbalance between calories consumed and calories expended. Contributing factors include increased consumption of fatty food and a decrease in physical activity due to the sedentary nature of work, changing modes of transport and urbanisation.

Management of childhood obesity

Supportive environments and communities are fundamental in shaping children's choices. They contribute towards making the healthier choice of foods and regular physical activity the easiest choice (accessible, available and affordable), and therefore help prevent obesity (3).

On an individual level, families can promote the limited intake of sugar and fat, increased consumption of fruit and vegetables, as well as legumes, whole grains and nuts, and regular engagement in physical activity (60 minutes a day for children and 150 minutes per week for adolescents). At a social level, it is important to support individuals in following the above recommendations through sustained professional and political commitment, and ensure that these options are affordable and easily accessible. The food industry can help to promote healthy diets by reducing the fat, sugar and salt content of processed foods and ensuring that these are available at an affordable price to all consumers, and by practising responsible marketing, especially those aimed at children and teenagers.

The WHO has taken several steps in the right direction (1), and the following are some examples:

- Global action plan for the prevention and control of noncommunicable diseases 2013–2020 (2013)

- The Political Declaration of the High Level Meeting of the United Nations General Assembly on the Prevention and Control of Non-communicable Diseases (2011)

- Setting up of a high-level Commission on Ending Childhood Obesity (ECHO) (2010)

- The WHO Global strategy on diet, physical activity and health (2004)

Table 15.2: Complications of obesity in children (3)

Physical complications	Social and emotional complications
• Type 2 diabetes – A manifestation of peripheral insulin resistance • Metabolic syndrome – Refers to a combination of high blood pressure, high blood sugar, high triglycerides, low HDL (good) • Cholesterol and excess abdominal fat – These enhance the risk of developing heart disease and diabetes • High cholesterol and high blood pressure • Asthma – Higher prevalence in obese children • Sleep disorders – OSA • Nonalcoholic fatty liver disease (NAFLD) – Can lead to scarring and liver damage • Early puberty or menstruation	• Low self-esteem and bullying • Behaviour and learning problems • Depression

Syllabus Mapping

Nutrition

- Be able to assess, diagnose and manage malnutrition, obesity and their complications

References and Further Reading

1. World Health Organisation. Global strategy on diet, physical activity and health: Childhood overweight and obesity. http://www.who.int/dietphysicalactivity/childhood/en/.

2. Public Health England. Child Obesity. http://www.noo.org.uk/NOO_about_obesity/child_obesity.

3. Gurnani M, Birken C, Hamilton J. Childhood Obesity: Causes, Consequences, and Management. *Pediatr Clin North Am* 2015; 62: 821–40. doi: 10.1016/j.pcl.2015.04.001

Chapter 16: A 2 year old girl with an irregular pupil and white reflex
Dr Neil Rogers

16

A 2 year old Asian girl, the daughter of non-consanguineous parents, had been born at full term by normal vaginal delivery after an uncomplicated pregnancy. She has recently arrived in the UK. During routine examination, it is noted that the left pupil is abnormal in shape and that the red reflex appears white from some angles. The rest of the physical examination is entirely normal. There is no family history of ocular or systemic disease. Retinal examination showed this appearance.

Image 16.1

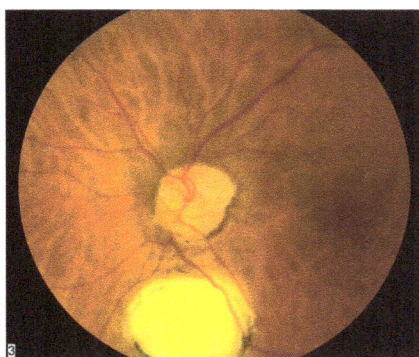

Image 16.2

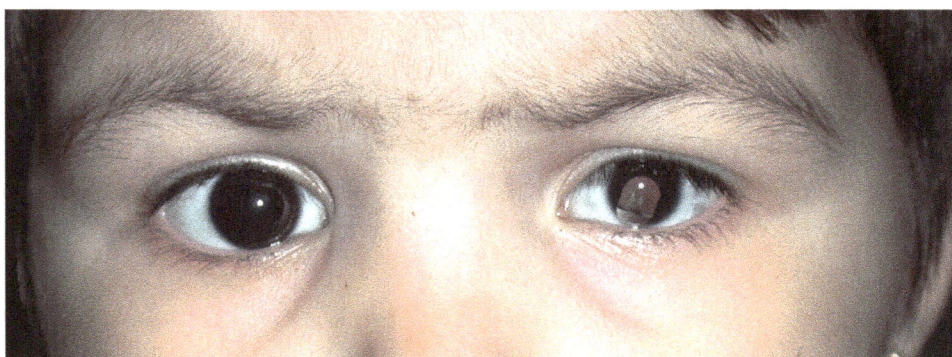

Investigations

Full blood count	normal
Urea and electrolytes	normal
TORCH screen	negative
Cardiac ultrasound	normal
Abdominal ultrasound	normal
Hearing test	normal

Q1. Which of the following is the most likely diagnosis?

Select one answer only

A. Choroideraemia
B. Coloboma
C. Congenital toxoplasmosis
D. Retinoblastoma
E. Tuberous sclerosis

Q2. Which of the following procedures is the next most important?

Select one answer only

A. MRI scan of the head
B. Refraction for spectacle prescription
C. Repeat renal ultrasound
D. Visually evoked potentials
E. Wood's lamp examination

Answers and Rationale

Q1.   B: Coloboma
Q2.   B: Refraction for spectacle prescription

The abnormally shaped pupil is a unilateral iris coloboma, and the retinal image is of a chorioretinal coloboma. In the absence of any other clinical findings, it is most likely to be isolated to the eye and not associated with any systemic features. Retinoblastoma would not cause an iris defect. Tuberous sclerosis may have associated retinal astrocytomas that are white, but will have no iris defect. Toxoplasmosis may cause retinal atrophic scars, but no iris abnormality. Choroideraemia shows retinal atrophic patches, but no iris defect.

In an eye with one anomaly, there are often other ocular abnormalities, including refractive error. In a child with an iris coloboma (the images also show a smaller corneal diameter and a lens notch), there is a high likelihood of a refractive error, which, if left uncorrected, would lead to amblyopia and strabismus. It is important to monitor the vision of these children and ensure that appropriate refractive correction is given and patching occurs if necessary. An MRI scan of the head is unlikely to be helpful in what appears to be an isolated coloboma. A repeat renal ultrasound might be appropriate in a condition such as aniridia, where there is a high risk of Wilms' tumour, but not for an isolated coloboma. Visual evoked potentials will not help with the visual prognosis, which appears to be good. Wood's lamp examination would only be relevant if tuberous sclerosis is suspected.

Coloboma is an ocular abnormality associated with a bewildering number of syndromes and gene mutations (1). Clinically, it is divided into isolated coloboma, those associated with other ocular abnormalities (e.g. cataract, microphthalmia, glaucoma), and those associated with systemic disease. Retinal detachment may occur in later life, and these children should remain under review. If the optic nerve and macula are not involved, the prognosis for good vision is excellent.

CHARGE syndrome (2) includes Coloboma, Heart defects, Choanal atresia, Retardation (of growth and/or development), and Genital and Ear abnormalities. It is an autosomal dominant condition, but most cases are sporadic. Approximately two thirds of cases are associated with mutations of the CHD7 gene on 8q12.

The differential diagnosis of leukocoria (a white light reflex) includes (3):

- Cataract
- Persistent hyperplastic primary vitreous (persistent fetal vasculature)
- Organised vitreous haemorrhage
- Retinoblastoma
- Retinal detachment
- Retrolental fibroplasia (stage 5 retinopathy of prematurity)
- Medulloepithelioma
- Giant retinal astrocytoma
- Norrie's syndrome

- Congenital toxoplasmosis
- Toxocariasis
- Coats' disease
- Leukaemic infiltration of the vitreous
- TB

Syllabus Mapping

Ophthalmology

- Be able to assess diagnose and manage visual impairment

- Be able to assess, diagnose and manage common ophthalmological conditions including glaucoma and papilloedema and know when to refer

References and Further Reading

1. Gregory-Evans CY, Williams MJ, Halford S, Gregory-Evans K. Ocular coloboma: A reassessment in the age of molecular neuroscience. J Med Genet 2004; 41: 881–891.

2. Sanlaville D, Verloes A. CHARGE syndrome: An update. Eur J Hum Genetics 2007; 15: 389–399.

3. Balmer A, Munier F. Differential diagnosis of leukocoria and strabismus. First presenting signs of retinoblastoma. Clinical Ophthalmology 2007; 1: 431–439.

Chapter 17: A teenage girl who took some tablets
Dr Robert Dinwiddie

17

A 15 year old girl presents to the emergency department at 4 pm with nausea and vomiting. She says that, at 8 am that morning, she had taken 20 adult paracetamol tablets. She is known to have expressed depressive feelings and suicidal thoughts on social media at various times during the previous 6 months.

On examination, she is conscious and alert and is normally grown and developed for her age. Her heart rate is 110/minute, respiratory rate 23/minute and blood pressure 115/85 mmHg. Her physical examination is otherwise normal. Baseline full blood count, electrolytes and liver function tests are normal. Her paracetamol level is subsequently reported as 105 mg/l.

Figure 17.1: Plasma concentrations for IV acetylcysteine treatment

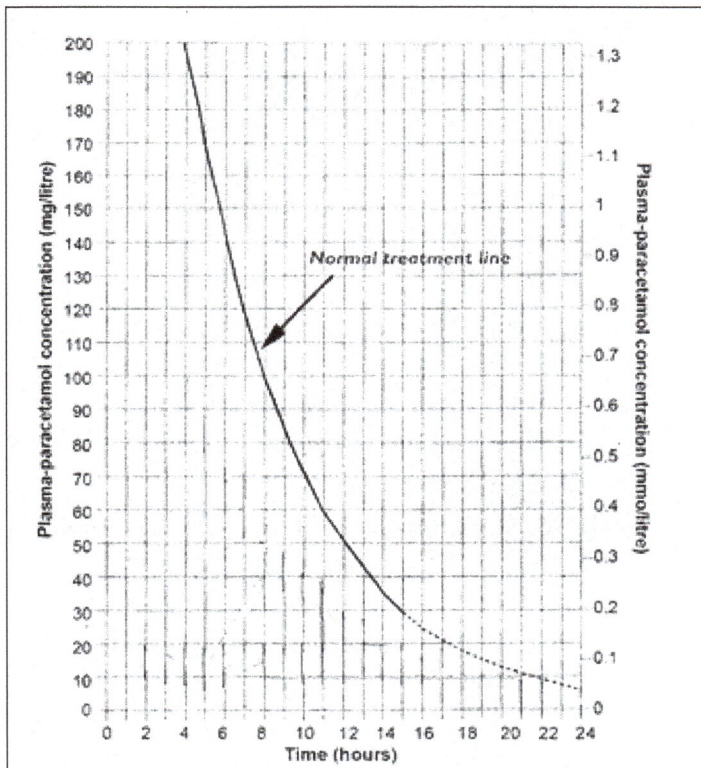

Acknowledgement to Therapeutics and Toxicolology Centre, Wales College of Medicine

Q1. Which of the following is the most appropriate action at this stage?

Select one answer only

A. Administration of activated charcoal
B. Admit, observe and repeat an examination of the paracetamol level in 4 hours
C. Gastric lavage
D. IV acetylcysteine
E. Refer for haemodialysis

Q2. Which of the following is the most frequent serious complication of paracetamol poisoning?

Select one answer only

A. Cerebral oedema
B. Gastric haemorrhage
C. Hepatic necrosis
D. Hypoglycaemia
E. Renal tubular necrosis

Answers and Rationale

Q1. **D: IV acetylcysteine**
Q2. **C: Hepatic necrosis**

Paracetamol (acetaminophen) is one of the most commonly used analgesics in children. In general use, it has an excellent safety profile and a better therapeutic index in children than in adults. Overdose in this age group does, however, occur due to chronic overuse by caregivers, accidental ingestion (particularly in young children) and deliberate overdose in adolescents. In the UK and the USA, deliberate paracetamol overdose has overtaken acute viral hepatitis as the most common cause of acute hepatic failure. It is also one of the leading indications for liver transplantation.

Paracetamol is the most frequently used agent for deliberate self-poisoning in UK adolescents. Ingestion of 150 mg/kg or more, taken acutely or spread out over a 24-hour period, can result in severe hepatocellular necrosis. The standard adult tablet size available in retail shops is 500 mg. In a young girl such as this, with an average body weight of 53 kg, ingestion of 16 such tablets would reach this level.

Paracetamol is metabolised in the liver (1), where the majority is conjugated to sulphate and glucuronide (which are non-toxic). Approximately 10% is metabolised into a toxic metabolite NAPQI; this occurs through the CYP450 system. In normal circumstances, NAPQI is conjugated with glutathione, which renders it inactive. When an overdose of 150 mg/kg or more is taken, the major pathways become saturated and excess amounts of paracetamol are presented to the CYP450 system for conjugation. All available glutathione is used up and toxic amounts of free NAPQI circulate, which – after 24 hours – results in acute hepatic necrosis (1). The damage is maximal at 3–4 days post ingestion.

Initial symptoms of paracetamol overdose include nausea and vomiting, which usually settles within 24 hours. Persistence beyond this time in combination with the onset of subcostal pain and tenderness usually indicates the development of acute hepatic necrosis (2). Plasma paracetamol concentration, measured after not less than 4 hours of ingestion, can be used to determine the need for more aggressive treatment. Initially, activated charcoal can be given but it is only useful within 1 hour of ingestion. Gastric lavage has also been used, but has been shown to be less effective than activated charcoal. The most effective treatment is with intravenous acetylcysteine (parvolex), especially if it can be started within 8 hours of ingestion. Figure 43.1 shows the treatment line based on plasma paracetamol concentration. If the paracetamol level exceeds the treatment line, then intravenous acetylcysteine should be started immediately. There is no point in waiting for a further repeat level 4 hours later. It is also recommended that those who have taken an excess of tablets spread over several hours should be treated with intravenous acetylcysteine regardless of the paracetamol concentration on admission. If there is likely to be a delay in the reporting of the paracetamol level in cases suspected of having ingested 150 mg/kg or more within the last 8–24 hours, then acetylcysteine should be commenced. It can be discontinued if the plasma concentration subsequently falls below the treatment line and if the patient is asymptomatic.

The most frequent serious complication of paracetamol poisoning is hepatic failure secondary to hepatic necrosis. This is treated with haemodialysis. Renal tubular necrosis also occurs but is less common. Other complications, including hypoglycaemia, cerebral oedema and gastric haemorrhage, are complications related to hepatic failure secondary to hepatocellular necrosis.

Apart from the physical treatments described, patients with deliberate paracetamol poisoning should be admitted to hospital for full emotional and psychological assessment, along with referrals to the appropriate supportive and mental health services for follow-up.

Syllabus mapping

Emergency Medicine including Accidents and Poisoning

- Be able to identify causes of poisoning and their presentation, know how to initiate appropriate management and be able to anticipate potential complications

References and Further Reading

1. Sandell J. Accidents and Emergencies. In: Gardiner M, Eisen S, Murphy C (eds). Training in Paediatrics. Oxford University Press: Oxford, 2009: 29–52.

2. Emergency treatment of poisoning. British National Formula for Children 2015–2016:754–755. Pharmpress

Chapter 18: A child with immunodeficiency and haemoptysis
Dr Rob Primhak

A 9 year old girl presents with a 6 month history of a tickly cough, sometimes productive of clear sputum, and 2 episodes of haemoptysis in the previous 24 hours. She has a history of a neck abscess, recurrent oral thrush and subsequent right upper lobe Staphylococcal pneumonia in infancy, with a persisting pneumatocele. This led to a diagnosis of hyper-IgE syndrome. She has been well since that time, until the current presentation, on prophylactic co-trimoxazole.

On examination, she is afebrile and in no respiratory distress. She has a central trachea, symmetrical percussion note but decreased air entry over the right upper lobe. Her chest x-rays are shown in the figures below.

Figure 18.1: Chest image

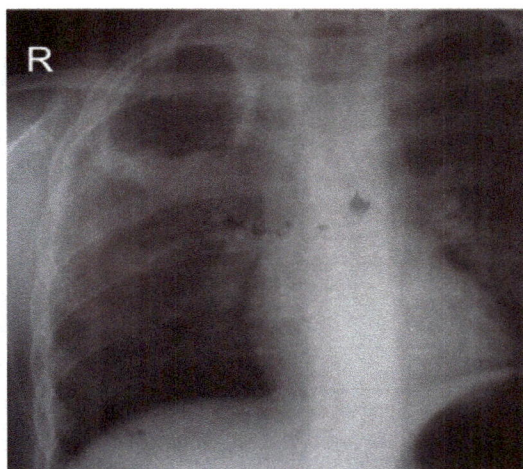

Figure 18.2: Chest image

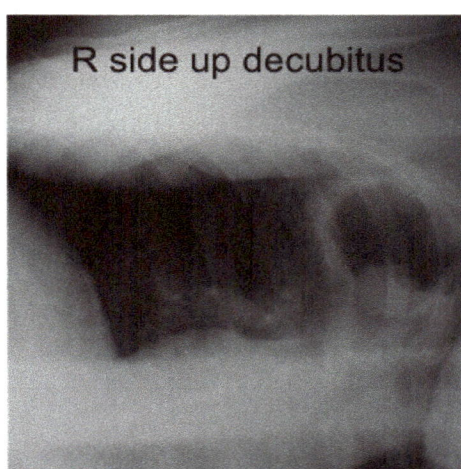

Q1. What is the most appropriate management?

Select <u>one</u> answer only

A. Flucloxacillin and clindamycin for 4 weeks
B. Rifampicin, isoniazid, pyrazinamide and ethambutol
C. Itraconazole
D. Diagnostic aspiration of the lesion
E. Right upper lobectomy

Q2. What is the likely cause of the recent problem?

Select <u>one</u> answer only

A. Aspergilloma
B. Candida infection
C. Invasive aspergillosis
D. Nontuberculous mycobacterial infection
E. Staphylococcal infection

Answers and Rationale

Q1.   E: Right upper lobectomy
Q2.   A: Aspergilloma

Hyper-IgE syndrome is an immune deficiency that has two varieties, the most common of the two rare disorders is a dominant form, due to a loss of function mutation in the signal transducer and activator of the transcription-3 (STAT3) gene. Classically, it causes mild dysmorphism (with coarse facies, a broad nasal bridge and prominent forehead) and eczema. Children affected by this type have a generalised susceptibility to infections, but a particular propensity to mucocutaneous candidiasis and indolent Staphylococcal infections. Staphylococcal pneumonia often leads to a pneumatocele, and unlike a Staphylococcal pneumatocele in an otherwise healthy individual, these pneumatoceles are generally persistent. Other features of dominant hyper-IgE syndrome are listed in the table below.

Table 18.1: Hyper-IgE syndrome due to STAT3 mutation
(Clinical features occurring in >75% of cases)

Immunologically mediated	Non-immunologically mediated
Newborn rash	Characteristic facies
Boils	Retained primary teeth
Recurrent pneumonias	Minimal trauma fractures
Pneumatoceles	Scoliosis >10 degrees
Eczema	Hyperextensibility
Mucocutaneous candidiasis	
Peak serum IgE >2000 IU/ml	
Eosinophilia	

A much rarer recessive form of the hyper-IgE syndrome has less physical manifestations, but also has marked immune dysfunction with a greater tendency to viral infections.

The symptoms in this case are typical of an aspergilloma (see below) and, while other diagnoses are possible, this is the best option. Pneumatoceles in hyper-IgE patients are particularly prone to aspergillus infection, causing a fungal ball in the cavity, known as an aspergilloma. The x-ray in this case is helpful, as it shows the mobile nature of the solid material within the pneumatocele, which would also be consistent with an aspergilloma. Of the other diagnostic options given, Staphylococcal infection would generally be a more severe and acute problem and usually affects lung tissue rather than cavities. Candidiasis is generally mucocutaneous rather than pulmonary. TB is not common in this condition and, again, would generally affect lung tissue. Atypical mycobacteria can infect hyper-IgE patients but generally in the bronchiectatic lung rather than cavities.

Antifungal treatment of an aspergilloma is rarely effective, and the very occasional reported cure has required years of therapy. Since there is a risk of life-threatening haemoptysis, the preferred option is to remove the pneumatocele; this generally involves a lobectomy (1).

Aspergillus (usually fumigatus, but occasionally other species) can cause three main conditions in the lung, which are very different.

Aspergilloma is a fungal ball developing in an existing cavity, usually a persisting pneumatocele or, in the case of adults, a TB cavity. The usual presenting symptoms are cough and haemoptysis. Aspergillus IgG titres are often elevated, but specific IgE titres are not, and skin tests are negative. Antifungal treatment of an aspergilloma is rarely effective, and the very occasional reported cure has required years of therapy. Expectant management may be appropriate if the patient is asymptomatic. There is a risk of life-threatening haemoptysis in symptomatic patients, and the only sure way of preventing this is to remove the pneumatocele, generally involving a lobectomy.

Allergic bronchopulmonary aspergillosis (ABPA) is an immune reaction to colonisation with aspergillus, typically seen in cystic fibrosis (CF) but occasionally in a severe asthmatic (2). In the CF patient, it causes a clinical deterioration with increased cough and wheeze, worsening pulmonary function, mucus plugging, and infiltrates appearing radiologically. Total IgE is raised (>1000) and specific IgE and IgG to aspergillus and positive immediate hypersensitivity on the skin test are present. Treatment is with systemic steroids and antifungals.

Invasive aspergillosis in the lung is a disease of bone marrow suppression or failure, typically seen in patients receiving chemotherapy or after bone marrow transplant (3). It presents as a severe pneumonia resistant to antibacterial treatment, with a high spiking fever and pulmonary infiltrates. The typical cavitation, with crescent and halo signs on the x-ray seen in adults, are less common in children. Diagnosis can be very difficult, as even bronchoalveolar lavage does not always detect the organism, which is largely intraparenchymal. Biopsy may be necessary to confirm the diagnosis. Treatment is with aggressive systemic antifungals, either using an azole such as voriconazole or with liposomal amphotericin.

Syllabus Mapping

Respiratory

- Be able to assess, diagnose and manage lower respiratory tract infections

Infection Immunity and Allergy

- Know the causes and common presentations of vulnerability to infection including primary/secondary immunodeficiency and when to refer

References

1. Regnard JF, Icard P, Nicolosi M, Spagiarri L, Magdeleinat P, Jauffret B et al. Aspergilloma: a series of 89 surgical cases. Annals of Thoracic Surgery 2000; 69: 898–903.

2. Walsh TJ, Anaisse EJ, Denning DW et al. Treatment of Aspergillosis: Clinical Practice Guidelines of the Infectious Diseases Society of America. Clin Infect Dis 2008; 46: 327–60.

3. Patterson K, Strek M. Allergic Bronchopulmonary Aspergillosis. Proc Am Thorac Soc 2010; 7: 237–44.

Chapter 19: A collapsed 72 hour old baby boy
Dr Robert Dinwiddie

(19)

A baby boy was born at term by normal delivery after an uneventful pregnancy. His birthweight was 3.5 kg. His appearance at birth was normal and he was sent to the postnatal ward with his mother to establish breastfeeding. At 72 hours of age, he is found in his cot pale, tachypnoeic and mottled. He responds poorly to stimulation and is difficult to rouse.

On examination, he is jaundiced, his chest is clinically clear and the heart sounds are normal. There is no hepatosplenomegaly. His tone is poor and he is generally hypotonic. Reflexes are present but reduced. His capillary refill time is 4 seconds. His bedside glucose is 3.1 mmol/l and capillary blood gases show a partially compensated metabolic acidosis. He is immediately transferred to the neonatal intensive care unit where he is intubated, ventilated and started on IV antibiotics.

Investigations

Blood

Haemoglobin	169 g/l
White cell count	15.3 x 10⁹/l
Neutrophils	9.3 x 10⁹/l
Lymphocytes	6.0 x 10⁹/l
Platelets	450 x 10⁹/l
PT	14 seconds (10–15)
APTT	45 seconds (22–45)
CRP	10 mg/l
Sodium	140 mmol/l
Potassium	4.0 mmol/l
Chloride	100 mmol/l
Urea	2.5 mmol/l
Creatinine	35 µmol/l
Total bilirubin	180 µmol/l
Ammonia	950 µmol/l (30–100)
Blood culture	awaited

Q1. Which of the following is the most likely diagnosis?

Select one answer only

A. Group B Streptococcal septicaemia
B. Haemorrhagic disease of the newborn
C. Ornithine transcarbamylase deficiency (urea cycle defect)
D. Transient hyperammonaemia of the newborn (THAN)
E. Hyperammonaemia-hyperinsulinism disorder

Q2. Which of the following management options will best improve his prognosis at this stage?

Select one answer only

A. 10% dextrose infusion
B. Exchange transfusion
C. Haemodialysis
D. IM vitamin K
E. Total IV feeding

Answers and Rationale

Q1. **C: Ornithine transcarbamylase deficiency (urea cycle defect)**
Q2. **C: Haemodialysis**

The history, clinical findings and laboratory results suggest that this baby is suffering from a urea cycle defect. Although the most frequent cause of collapse at this age would be neonatal septicaemia, this is less likely due to the normal white blood cell count and CRP levels. Although plasma ammonia can be elevated in neonatal sepsis, it would not approach the levels seen here. It is, however, important to measure ammonia levels in any collapsed neonate, particularly if there is clinical evidence of an encephalopathy. Samples should ideally reach the laboratory within 1 hour. If this is not possible, the plasma should be kept on ice until the measurement is made. Otherwise, falsely elevated levels can occur. Apart from urea cycle disorders, neonatal hyperammonaemia occurs for a number of other reasons. These include Transient hyperammonaemia of the newborn (THAN), mainly seen in preterm infants (particularly those on parenteral nutrition) and in organic acidaemias such as propionic acidaemia and methylmalonic acidaemia. It is also seen in hyperammonaemia-hyperinsulinism, which is an autosomal dominant disorder caused by mutations on the glutamate dehydrogenase gene. This enzyme deficiency can result in severe neonatal hypoglycaemia, but only in mildly elevated ammonia levels (<400 μmol/l), which are not seen in this case (1, 2).

THAN can be differentiated from urea cycle enzyme deficiencies (UCEDs) on a number of clinical grounds. Thirty-three neonates with THAN had a mean gestational age at birth of 35.1 weeks versus 39.6 weeks in 13 patients with UCEDs. Mean birthweight was 2.23 kg versus 3.34 kg. All but 1 patient with THAN had respiratory symptoms (with a mean time of onset of 3.9 hours) but only 8 of the UCED patients had these signs, none before 30 hours, with a mean time of onset of 71.5 hours. Mean plasma ammonia concentration in THAN patients was 1871 μmol/l versus 973 μmol/l in those with UCEDs (3).

The urea cycle (also known as the ornithine cycle) is a multi-step, principally hepatic-based, metabolic pathway in which the nitrogen content of excess dietary amino acids is converted from highly toxic ammonia to urea, which is then excreted via the kidneys. A number of inborn metabolism errors involving the urea cycle are described. They are all inherited as autosomal recessives except for ornithine transcarbamylase deficiency, which is inherited as an X-linked trait. The family history in ornithine transcarbamylase deficiency cases often includes previous early deaths of male infants in the neonatal period. Each urea cycle defect presents in its most severe form with acute collapse and encephalopathy during the neonatal period.

Children with urea cycle defects can also present with milder versions at any time during childhood and occasionally even into adult life (1). Specific enzyme defects causing hyperammonaemia include N-acetylglutamate synthase deficiency, carbamoyl phosphate synthetase deficiency, ornithine transcarbamylase deficiency, various forms of citrullinaemia, argininosuccinic aciduria, argininaemia, and hyperornithinaemia-hyperammonaemia-hypercitrullinuria (HHH) syndrome (1, 2). Ornithine transcarbamylase takes the molecule carbamoyl phosphate and combines it with ornithine to make citrulline. When the enzyme is deficient, excess carbamoyl phosphate is converted into orotic acid. This leads to an elevation of plasma ammonia, decreased blood urea and increased serum and urinary orotic acid levels. When the diagnosis of ornithine transcarbamylase deficiency is suspected, elevated plasma glutamine and alanine with low citrulline in the presence of elevated urine orotic acid levels is diagnostic. The enzyme itself can be assayed in hepatocytes and in duodenal mucosal cells (1, 2).

Treatment of acute hyperammonaemia is multimodal. This includes maximising fluid intake to ensure that adequate renal function is maintained. Calorie requirements are principally met by an intravenous glucose infusion in order to minimise protein catabolism from primarily protein sources. A concurrent insulin infusion may be required to control any associated hyperglycaemia. Arginine is useful in reducing plasma ammonia levels, particularly in ornithine transcarbamylase deficiency. Other drugs ('ammonia scavengers') that reduce plasma ammonia levels include sodium benzoate and sodium phenylbutyrate. These agents contain significant amounts of sodium, so should be used with care, especially where there is evidence of congestive heart failure or renal insufficiency. They are also used in the long-term management of these conditions. Haemodialysis is the most effective and rapid way to reduce acutely elevated ammonia levels and to improve the long-term prognosis. Current guidelines suggest that this is started when neonatal ammonia levels exceed 250 µmol/l in the presence of encephalopathic symptoms (2).

Initial mortality among affected male infants in the neonatal period is reported as up to 50% (2). The long-term intellectual and developmental outcomes in survivors are directly related to the severity and duration of the initial hyperammonaemia. Liver transplantation in the first year of life, preferably carried out after 3 months of age, can be curative (2).

Syllabus Mapping

Metabolic

- Know the biochemical features of metabolic diseases and be able to undertake and interpret relevant metabolic investigations

- Have a good understanding of the clinical presentation and prognosis of metabolic diseases

References and Further Reading

1. Grompe M. Disorders of amino acid metabolism. In: McIntosh N, Helms P, Smyth RL, Logan S (eds). Forfar and Arneil's Textbook of Pediatrics, 7th edition. Churchill-Livingstone Elsevier: 2008:1052–1067.

2. Haberle J, Boddaert N, Burlina A et al. Suggested guidelines for the diagnosis and management of urea cycle disorders. Orphanet Journal of Rare Diseases 2012; 7:32.

3. Hudak ML, Jones MD Jr, Brusilow SW. Differentiation of transient hyperammonemia of the newborn and urea cycle defects by clinical presentation. Journal of Pediatrics 1985; 107: 712–719.

Chapter 20: A 7 year old boy with a heart murmur
Dr Andrew Boon

This ECG was recorded from a 7 year old boy who was born in Sudan and has recently moved with his parents to the UK. His parents report that he was first noted to have a heart murmur at 6 weeks of age, but he has not undergone surgery.

Image 20.1: ECG

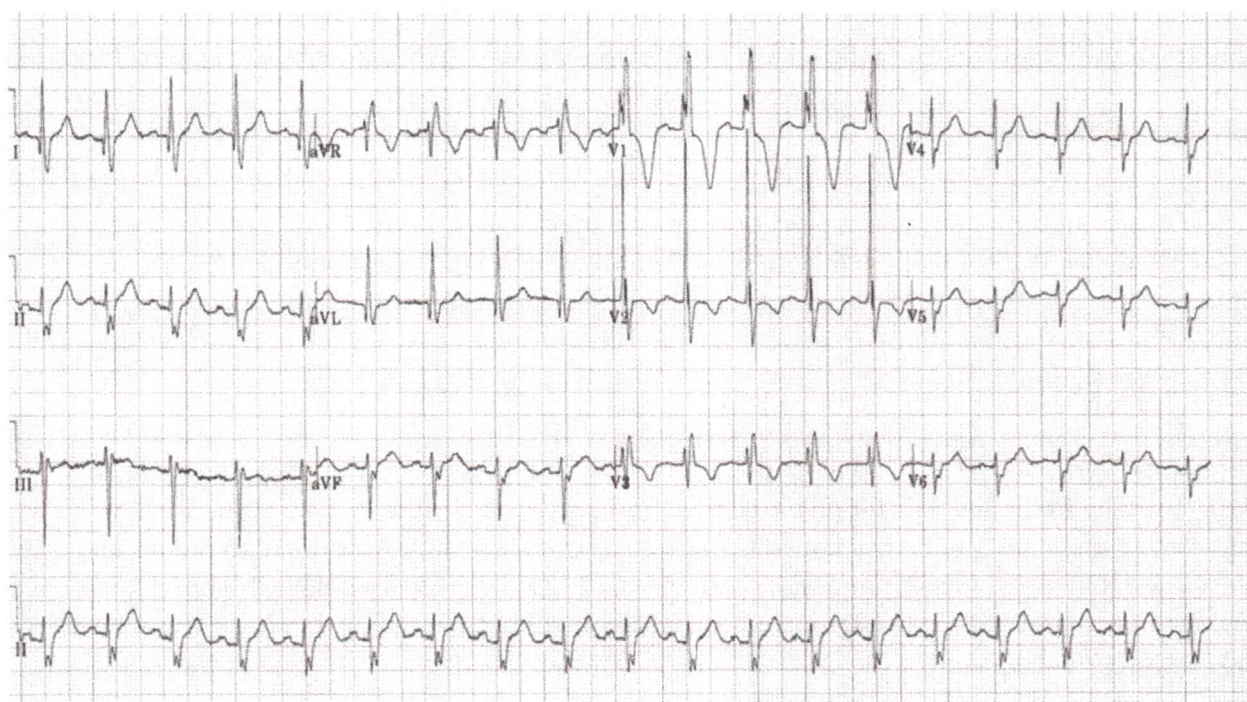

25.0mm/sec   10.0mm/mV

Q1. Which of the following abnormalities are seen on the ECG?

Select <u>two</u> answers from the list below

A. Abnormal ST segment
B. Abnormal T waves
C. Delta waves
D. Left axis deviation
E. Left ventricular hypertrophy
F. P pulmonale
G. Prolonged QT interval
H. Right axis deviation
I. Right bundle branch block
J. Right ventricular hypertrophy

Q2. What is the most likely underlying cardiac abnormality?

Select <u>one</u> answer only

A. Atrioventricular septal defect
B. Ostium secundum atrial septal defect
C. Patent ductus arteriosus
D. Primary pulmonary hypertension
E. Ventricular septal defect

Answers and Rationale

Q1. **D: Left axis deviation**
I: Right bundle branch block
Q2. **A: Atrioventricular septal defect**

The paediatric ECG has an important place in the investigation of a child with a heart murmur, and is widely available. It is important to follow a structured approach to the interpretation of an ECG (see below) (1, 2). Although most ECG machines will now provide an automated analysis of the ECG, it is important to remember that this is usually programmed for analysis of the adult ECG and may therefore misinterpret the paediatric ECG (3).

In following a structured approach, you will be able to quickly rule out many of the possibilities and should be able to identify that this ECG shows left axis deviation with right bundle branch block. More specifically, the mean frontal QRS on this occasion gives a superior axis (between -1 and -180 degrees), which is always abnormal.

There are only a few structural congenital cardiac abnormalities where the ECG will provide a very likely diagnosis. However, the superior axis and right bundle branch block seen in this ECG are the typical findings seen in a child with an atrioventricular septal defect (4). Most children with this diagnosis will undergo corrective cardiac surgery at 3 to 6 months of age to prevent the development of pulmonary hypertension.

An ostium secundum atrial septal defect (an uncomplicated septal defect without associated valvular abnormality) is typically associated with right axis deviation and right bundle branch block. A ventricular septal defect with a significant shunt may cause biventricular hypertrophy, or progress to pulmonary hypertension. A patent arterial duct is not associated with an ECG abnormality unless the child develops pulmonary hypertension. Pulmonary hypertension causes right ventricular hypertrophy often associated with peaked P waves (P pulmonale).

Box 20.2: A suggested structured approach in ECG interpretation

1. *Examine the P waves.*

Is each QRS complex preceded by a P wave and is the PR interval constant and of normal duration? Are the P waves peaked (P pulmonale)? In this ECG, the P waves are normal (best seen in leads II and V1) which excludes answer G: P pulmonale.

2. *Determine the heart rate.*

One should next look at the heart rate (obviously not possible in this ECG). With the usual paper speed of 25 mm/ seconds, each small square represents 0.04 seconds (40 milliseconds) and each big square 0.2 seconds. The rate can be calculated by dividing 300 by the number of large squares between consecutive R waves.

3. *Assess the mean frontal QRS axis.*

The simplest way of estimating the QRS axis is to find a lead with a roughly equiphasic QRS complex. In the ECG shown, this is lead II. The QRS axis will be at 90 degrees to this – thus, either -30 degrees or +150 degrees. Since the QRS deflection is upward in aVL, the axis must be -30 degrees, i.e. a superior axis or left axis deviation.

4. *Check the shape of the QRS complexes.*

Are the complexes widened? Is there an abnormal pattern of conduction? Pre-excitation results in a delta wave (an upslur on the R wave). Right bundle branch block produces an RSR pattern in V1 (seen in this case), whereas left bundle branch block produces a broadened QS or rS shape in V1.

5. *Check the size (amplitude) of the QRS complexes.*

The amplitude of QRS complexes indicates the voltage produced. High voltages are seen in ventricular hypertrophy. Right ventricular hypertrophy produces tall R waves in right sided chest leads (V4R and V1) and deep S waves in left chest leads (V5 and V6). Left ventricular hypertrophy produces tall R waves in the left chest leads and deep S waves in the right sided leads.

6. *Check the QT interval.*

The QT interval is the interval from the start of the Q wave to the end of the T wave. It varies with heart rate and is usually corrected for this using Bazett's formula to give the QTc. QTc = measured QT / √RR interval. The RR interval is 60/heart rate. For children over 6 months, the QTc should be less than 0.44 seconds.

7. *Check the ST segment.*

The ST segment is normally isoelectric. Elevation or depression is in relation to the TP segment.

8. *Look at the T waves.*

The T waves change with the child's age. For the first week, the T waves are upright in all the chest leads. After the first week, the T waves become inverted over the right chest leads until around the age of 8 years, when they become upright. Tall, peaked T waves are seen in hyperkalaemia and LVH. Flat T waves occur in hypokalaemia, pericarditis and with digoxin.

Syllabus Mapping

Cardiology

- Be able to assess, diagnose and manage murmurs, chest pain, palpitations, cardiac arrhythmias and syncope.

- Understand investigation of cardiac diseases e.g. ECG, ECHO, catheterisation and their appropriate selection in diagnosis and management.

References and Further Reading

1. Price A, Kaski J. How to use the paediatric ECG. Arch Dis Child Educ Pract Ed 2014; 99: 53-60.

2. Archer A, Barnes N. Cardiology. In: Gardiner M, Eisen S, Murphy C (eds). Training in Paediatrics. Oxford University Press: Oxford, 2009: 77-92.

3. Dickinson DF. The normal ECG in childhood and adolescence. Heart 2005; 91: 1626-1630.

4. Kitchener DJ. In: McIntosh N, Helms P, Smyth R, Logan S (eds). Forfar and Arneil's Textbook of Paediatrics, 7th edition. Churchill Livingstone: Edinburgh, 2008; ch21: 743-799.

Chapter 21: An infant with hypotonia, developmental delay and small hands and feet (21)
Dr Robert Dinwiddie

A 4 month old boy is referred because of "floppiness", poor feeding and faltering growth. He was born at term of normal birthweight after an uneventful pregnancy. On examination, he has a mild degree of generalised hypotonia, his reflexes are all present but weak. He is noted to have dysmorphic features, including almond-shaped eyes, a narrow nasal bridge and a thin upper lip with a downturned mouth.

Physical examination is otherwise normal except for a small penis and testes.

Q1. Which of the following is the most likely diagnosis?

Select <u>one</u> answer only

A. Angelman syndrome
B. Congenital myotonic dystrophy
C. Fetal alcohol syndrome
D. Prader-Willi syndrome
E. Spinal muscular atrophy

Q2. Which of the following is most likely to occur in children with this condition?

Select <u>one</u> answer only

A. Cardiomyopathy
B. Poor weight gain during early childhood
C. Progressive respiratory failure
D. Treatment resistant seizures
E. Sleep disordered breathing

Q3. Which is most likely to require replacement during adolescence?

Select <u>one</u> answer only

A. Growth hormone
B. Insulin-like growth factor (IGF)
C. Insulin
D. Thyroid stimulating hormone
E. Thyroxine

Answers and Rationale

Q1.   **D: Prader-Willi syndrome**
Q2.   **E: Sleep disordered breathing**
Q3.   **A: Growth hormone**

The diagnostic conundrum here is not especially difficult. The causes of hypotonia (floppiness) in babies should be well rehearsed by most candidates. In clinical practice, it is helpful to split the children into 2 groups: those who are floppy and weak (these children have a primary nerve; spinal muscular atrophy) or muscle (muscular dystrophies) problem. Those who are floppy but remain relatively strong often have central hypotonia, which is often due to a syndromic cause (Down syndrome and Prader-Willi syndrome) (1).

The distractors offered are all important conditions in their own right though, and understanding why the question-writer has included them is helpful in answering the question. It is good exam technique to look at the pattern of conditions included in the answer stem for this type of question. Even if you think you know the correct answer in a 'single best answer' question, carefully going through the options can help to confirm that you are right.

Angelman syndrome is genetically related to Prader-Willi syndrome, as both conditions result from microdeletions of chromosome 15q11.2-13 (2). Deletion of the *paternal* copy leads to Prader-Willi syndrome. It does not result in hypotonia but its presence in the answer list should make you feel more confident that Prader-Willi syndrome is the correct answer. Fetal alcohol syndrome is incorrect because although there are dysmorphic facial features, including micrognathia, epicanthic folds, a low nasal bridge, small philtrum and a thin upper lip, hypotonia is not a classical feature. Congenital myotonic dystrophy and spinal muscular atrophy type 1 are both examples of 'floppy weak' (peripheral hypotonia). Neither is associated with dysmorphic features in infancy, although there may be myopathic facies in children with congenital myotonic dystrophy and tongue fasciculation in children with spinal muscular atrophy type 1.

Prader-Willi syndrome is a rare condition that affects approximately 1 in 15,000 to 1 in 22,000 children born in the UK. Males and females are equally affected. The recurrence rate for the most frequent genetic type (involving the paternal microdeletion described above) is less than 1%. It presents in early infancy with hypotonia, feeding difficulties due to a reduced sucking reflex, and developmental delay. Physical features include small hands and feet, hypogonadism and facial dysmorphism, including almond-shaped eyes, a narrow nasal bridge, a thin upper lip and downturned mouth. Hypogonadism includes cryptorchidism, undescended testes and a micropenis, which are problems for boys; girls also have underdeveloped genitalia.

After the first year of life, the more classic symptoms of insatiable appetite and obesity increasingly develop. Children with Prader-Willi syndrome can tolerate larger amounts of food than normal and have a reduced metabolic rate. This, in conjunction with reduced muscle tone and the fact that they are less physically active than their peers, increases the risk of obesity as well as the development of type 2 diabetes later in life. Moderate intellectual impairment and developmental delay leads to learning difficulties in school-age years. Behavioural difficulties including temper tantrums and manipulative behaviour, especially in relation to eating, are frequent, although some children are described as "affectionate, kind and caring".

Infants and children with Prader-Willi syndrome also have problems with the central control of breathing. In infancy, this can be improved by the use of supplemental oxygen (3). This problem continues throughout childhood but, with increasing age, obstructive sleep apnoea (OSA) as secondary to obesity becomes an additional problem. This can result in daytime somnolence, which further decreases the time spent in physical activity. Disturbed nocturnal sleep patterns can also impair daytime behaviour and cognitive abilities. Treatment is with non-invasive ventilation (NIV) or continuous positive airway pressure (CPAP), if tolerated, and adenotonsillectomy to improve the airways in selected cases. Polysomnographic screening for sleep-related breathing disorders is recommended on an annual basis.

Hypogonadism leads to a high incidence of undescended testes in boys, which requires orchidopexy. Puberty in both sexes is delayed in onset and may not be fully completed. Facial and pubic hair is scanty or absent and, in males, the voice may not break. Most females have primary or secondary amenorrhoea and are infertile, although a few successful pregnancies have been reported. This lack of sex hormones, which is thought to be due to hypothalamic dysfunction, also predisposes one to osteoporosis in later life.

Growth impairment due to growth hormone deficiency previously led to short stature, but this can now be treated using growth hormone replacement therapy. Growth hormone therapy also improves muscle tone and mass, which can result in greater physical activity and thus reduce the risk of obesity. Patients with Prader-Willi syndrome have decreased sensitivity to pain such that significant injuries, even bone fractures, can go unrecognised. Decreased abdominal pain sensation can lead to the late diagnosis of conditions such as acute appendicitis. Easy bruising is another important clinical feature.

Life expectancy for patients with Prader-Willi syndrome is reduced but improving with time. It is hypothesised that, for a variety of reasons, premature ageing occurs in this condition. Recently, full clinical details of 12 patients with Prader-Willi syndrome over the age of 50 years have been described (4).

Syllabus Mapping

Genetics and Dysmorphology

- Be able to diagnose and manage common genetic and dysmorphological conditions and make appropriate referrals

References and Further Reading

1. Jain RK, Jayawant S. Evaluation of the floppy infant. Paediatrics and Child Health 2011; 21(11): 495–500.

2. Smith N. A teenager with an imprinting disorder. In: Royal College of Paediatrics and Child Health. Clinical cases for MRCPCH Theory and Science. London, 2014: 81–84.

3. Urquhart DS, Gulliver T, Williams G, Harris MA, Nyunt O, Suresh S. Central sleep-disordered breathing and the effects of oxygen therapy in infants with Prader-Will syndrome. Arch Dis Child 2013; 98: 592–595.

4. Sinnema M, Schrander-Stumpel CT, Maaskant MA, Boer H, Curfs LM. Aging in Prader-Willi syndrome: Twelve persons over the age of 50 years. Am J Med Genet A 2012; 158: 1326–36.

Chapter 22: An 11 year old girl with delayed puberty
Dr Robert Dinwiddie

22

An 11 year old girl is referred with short stature and delayed puberty. Over the previous year, it was noted that her height velocity was not keeping pace with her peers' despite both of her parents being tall with adult heights on the 90th centiles respectively for males and females. On examination, her height was 133 cm (0.5th centile). She was noted to have wide spaced nipples; breast development was stage 1 and pubic hair stage 2. She has cubitus valgus and hyperconvex fingernails.

Q1. Which of the following is the most likely diagnosis?

Select one answer only

A.   Constitutional delayed puberty
B.   Growth hormone deficiency
C.   Hypothyroidism
D.   Noonan syndrome
E.   Turner syndrome (TS)

Q2. Which investigation would be most likely to confirm the underlying diagnosis?

Select one answer only

A.   Array comparative genomic hybridisation (array CGH)
B.   Fluorescent in situ hybridisation (FISH)
C.   Karyotyping
D.   MR brain
E.   Thyroid function tests

Q3. Which treatment is most likely to prevent a complication?

Select one answer only

A.   Growth hormone
B.   Laparoscopic gonadectomy
C.   Oestrogen therapy
D.   Penicillin prophylaxis
E.   Thyroxine

Answers and Rationale

Q1.   **E: Turner syndrome (TS)**
Q2.   **C: Karyotyping**
Q3.   **C: Oestrogen therapy**

This girl has Turner syndrome (TS), one of the most common dysmorphic syndromes seen in this age group. She has a typical history and a number of the most frequently observed dysmorphic features. Delayed puberty can also occur for constitutional reasons and due to growth hormone deficiency, but these are not associated with dysmorphism. Similarly, while there is an increased incidence of hypothyroidism in TS, it is not the primary diagnosis in this case. While Noonan syndrome has several clinical features in common with TS, these children have hypertelorism and right-sided cardiac lesions that are not present in this case.

TS is a condition affecting about 1 in 2,500 live births in the UK as well as a significant number of early miscarriages. As many as 15% of spontaneous miscarriages in the UK have the 45X TS karyotype. The recurrence risk for parents who have one affected daughter is estimated to be 1.4% (1). TS presents at all ages, including prenatally. Severely affected fetuses can present with non-immune hydrops. Other features detectable on a prenatal ultrasound include raised nuchal translucency, horseshoe kidneys and left sided cardiac lesions. In the neonatal period, a number of typical dysmorphic features are seen.

These include webbing of the neck, low posterior hairline, 'shield' chest, widely spaced nipples, oedema of the hands and feet, a high arched palate and left sided cardiac lesions, including coarctation of the aorta and a bicuspid aortic valve. Affected infants can also have an increased carrying angle (cubitus valgus), short fourth metacarpals and hyperconvex nails (2). Ptosis and strabismus become evident with increasing age. As many as 60% of affected patients have renal tract anomalies, including horseshoe kidneys and duplex ureters, although this does not usually impair renal function.

Hypertension is more common than normal at all ages and should be screened for at regular intervals. A small percentage of TS patients have a mosaicism including Y chromosome material. These patients have a high risk of developing gonadoblastoma and, for them, laparoscopic gonadectomy is recommended as a preventative measure. Karyotyping is essential to identify this group.

A variety of genetic mechanisms can result in TS. The most common is absence of the paternal X chromosome accounting for approximately 60% of cases. At least 10% of cases are due to mosaicism. Much less frequently, partial absence of maternal X chromosome material and ring chromosomes result in TS. Genomic imprinting is seen in other conditions, such as Prader-Willi syndrome, but not in TS. Ring X chromosomes do occur in TS but are rare.

Array CGH has rapidly replaced the use of karyotyping for the investigation of most genetic disorders. Array CGH can detect genomic deletions or duplications with far greater sensitivity (>100 times) than can be achieved by chromosome analysis using light microscopy. It has several important limitations though. Array CGH cannot detect balanced chromosome rearrangements (e.g. translocations or inversions), low frequency mosaicism (< 30% abnormal cells) and polyploidy. Karyotyping is still the preferred method of testing for suspected Down (+21), Edwards (+18), Patau (+13) or Klinefelter (47,XXY) syndromes or TS (45,X).

TS may present later, as in this case, with late onset puberty, amenorrhoea and delayed secondary sexual characteristics. Ovarian dysgenesis is a typical feature. Pubic hair develops normally. Growth failure may not be apparent earlier in life, especially if the affected person has tall parents. Growth charts for girls with TS are readily available. If therapy with the growth hormone is started before the epiphyses are fused, then significant gains in final height are achievable. However, short stature in itself is not likely to lead to a complication.

Oestrogen therapy can be started at 12–15 years of age and facilitates breast development, as well as improves bone density and psychological maturation (3). Osteoporosis, which can be seen even in late childhood, contributes to an increased incidence of scoliosis in this age group. In the longer term, it significantly increases the risk of pathological fractures. Patients with TS usually have an IQ that is within the normal range but specific difficulties with visuospatial perception are not uncommon.

Most adults with TS are infertile due to ovarian dysgenesis, but they are however suitable candidates for in vitro fertilisation using donated ova. There is a higher incidence than normal of hypothyroidism due to autoimmune thyroiditis, and regular monitoring for this problem is recommended. Life expectancy for patients with TS can be reduced due to the risk of aortic dissection and an increased incidence of cardiovascular events. With the advent of multidisciplinary clinical teams, which focus especially on TS, these complications should become less frequent.

Syllabus Mapping

Genetics and Dysmorphology

- Be able to diagnose and manage common genetic and dysmorphological conditions and make appropriate referrals

References and Further Reading

1. Larizza D, Danesino C, Maraschio P, Caramanga C, Klersy C, Calcaterra V. Familial incidence of Turner syndrome: Casual event or increased risk? J Pediatr Endocrinol Metab 2011; 24: 223-5.

2. Elmslie F, Hanson H, Baple E. Genetics. In: Gardiner M, Eisen S, Murphy C (eds). Training in Paediatrics. Oxford University Press: Oxford, 2009: 247-268.

3. Kelnar CJH, Butler GE. Endocrine gland disorders and disorders of growth and puberty. In: McIntosh N, Helms P, Smyth R, Logan S (eds). Forfar and Arneil's Textbook of Pediatrics, 7th edition. Churchill Livingstone: Edinburgh, 2008: 409-512.

Chapter 23: A 4 year old with an abdominal mass
Dr Phoebe Sneddon, Dr Martin Hewitt

(23)

A 4 year old girl presents with a 3 week history of lethargy and abdominal pain. She has had episodic high temperatures and was not eating. She is passing small amounts of urine and has not had her bowels open for 5 days.

Examination showed her to be miserable, pale and sitting quietly on her mother's knee. She had palpable lymph nodes in the left upper and lower cervical area and obvious ecchymosis on her abdomen and limbs. Her temperature was 38.5°C, her blood pressure 130/85 mmHg and heart rate 110/minute. Auscultation revealed normal heart sounds and there was reduced air entry on the left lung base. Examination of the abdomen identified a mass on the right side, which extended from the costal margin to the iliac crest.

Investigations

Blood

Haemoglobin	85 g/l
White cell count	12.5 x 10^9/l
Platelets	18 x 10^9/l
Sodium	137 mmol/l
Potassium	4.3 mmol/l
Urea	6.2 mmol/l
Creatinine	31 mmol/l

Q1. Which of the following investigations is most likely to suggest the diagnosis?

Select one answer only

A.   Bone marrow aspirate
B.   Serum alpha-fetoprotein
C.   Serum Cancer Antigen 125 (CA 125)
D.   Serum lactate dehydrogenase
E.   Urinary catecholamines

Q2. Which of the following laboratory investigations will suggest metastatic disease?

Select one answer only

A.   Bone marrow aspirate
B.   CA 125
C.   Clotting studies
D.   Serum lactate dehydrogenase
E.   Urinary catecholamines

Answers and Rationale

Q1.   **E: Urinary catecholamines**
Q2.   **A: Bone marrow aspirate**

This history and examination is consistent with a diagnosis of neuroblastoma – abdominal mass with fevers without cause, left sided lymph nodes (Virchow's node) and evidence of marrow failure. Neuroblastoma is a tumour of sympathetic neural tissue and therefore produces excessive amounts of catecholamines (dopamine, adrenaline and noradrenaline) along with their breakdown products (vanillylmandelic acid and homovanillic acid). Although a biopsy sample is needed for confirmation, the raised catecholamines will 'suggest' the diagnosis. A bone marrow aspirate rarely includes the neuroblastoma cells and so could not 'suggest' the diagnosis, but it would confirm marrow failure from metastatic disease. Alpha-fetoprotein is raised in hepatoblastoma and CA 125 in ovarian carcinomas. LDH is a non-specific test of increased white blood cell activity. Neuroblastoma classically spreads to bone and bone marrow.

Solid tumours in children can present in a multitude of ways depending upon their location and size. Many such tumours can present with an obvious mass, which may be painful or inhibit function, but others may be located in deeper tissue and may not be evident until they are large or metastatic.

Those malignant tumours that arise in the abdomen can grow to a considerable size before they are recognised, although the age of the patient may influence the pattern of presentation. The identification of a mass at any site requires investigations to firstly determine its nature and, secondly, identify its extent and stage. Imaging has a major role in both characterising the mass and advising on the most appropriate route for biopsy. The identification of a solid malignant tumour must be made from histological and, where appropriate, cytogenetic analysis, as there are so many sub-types and rare variants that could require differing treatment protocols.

Neuroblastoma in the 2 to 5 years olds is predominantly an abdominal condition (about 75% of patients with this diagnosis) but as it arises from tissue making the sympathetic chain, the tumour can occur anywhere from behind the eye down to the pelvis. Most children in this age group present with metastatic disease and the extent of this can be identified by an MIBG scan that will show bone metastases. MIBG is a radiolabelled precursor of norepinephrine that is taken up by any neuroblastoma cell in the body, wherever it may be. The common sites of spreading are bone marrow (creating pancytopaenia), orbit and bone (proptosis and orbital bruising) and the left supraclavicular lymph nodes (Virchow's node). Consequently, clinical examination can identify metastatic disease at presentation. Increased production of catecholamines may lead to hypertension. An indication of the diagnosis comes from the detection of catecholamines on a 'spot urine' sample, which may provide a result before biopsy is undertaken.

The newborn with a neuroblastoma may present with massive abdominal distension, sometimes sufficient to interfere with normal delivery or subsequent breathing or feeding. Scanning may show massive hepatic enlargement along with a suprarenal mass, which fits the description of Stage IV S disease – a localised tumour with the involvement of skin, liver or bone only. Cytogenetic analysis of biopsy materials may demonstrate single copies of the oncogene, MYCN, and this imparts a favourable prognosis. Increased copies of the MYCN gene are usually seen in children with stage IV disease and who require more intensive treatment (1).

A number of other tumours may present with an abdominal mass. A child with a nephroblastoma (Wilms' tumour) is often well and the mass is found incidentally. Hypertension is present in about 25% of patients and haematuria in 15%. Assessment of the abdominal mass is undertaken with USS and an MRI while pulmonary metastases are assessed with a computer tomography (CT). Biopsy is needed to confirm the diagnosis and identify adverse pathological features. Treatment requires chemotherapy and nephrectomy. Radiotherapy is required in high stages of the disease and to treat metastases.

The child with a hepatoblastoma usually presents with anorexia, lethargy and hepatic enlargement. A massively raised AFP is invariably found. The condition commonly presents in the first 2 years of life and rarely in children over 5 years of age. They can be associated with a number of syndromes, including familial adenomatous polyposis (FAP) and Beckwith-Wiedemann. The disease usually occurs as a single mass arising from the liver. As with other solid tumours, biopsy and imaging are needed to confirm the diagnosis. The tumour is usually chemotherapy-sensitive, but surgery is needed for a cure. A liver transplant may be necessary if the tumour occupies the area around the porta hepatis or remains extensive after initial chemotherapy.

B-cell non-Hodgkin lymphomas arise from mesenteric lymph nodes. The child usually has a short history of lethargy, anorexia and abdominal distension. These tumours grow rapidly and they are very responsive to chemotherapy. Consequently, this means that these patients are at a high risk of tumour lysis syndrome at the induction of chemotherapy – a rapid rise in potassium, phosphate and purines (adenosine and guanosine). The long-term survival for these patients on current protocols is extremely good. Hodgkin lymphoma usually presents with cervical or inguinal lymphadenopathy and subsequent examination may identify hepatosplenomegaly. The triad of night sweats, weight loss and fever indicate the need for more intensive treatment (2).

Rhabdomyosarcomas arise in the soft tissues in the abdomen and pelvis, with the bladder, prostate and biliary tree as recognised sites. Presenting symptoms will vary due to the site. There are 4 main histological subtypes, but embryonal and alveolar are the ones most commonly seen in paediatric practice with the former usually in younger children and the latter in adolescents. Systemic treatment with chemotherapy needs to be supported by locally directed therapy – surgery or radiotherapy – and the site of the disease will suggest the most appropriate option (3).

Germ cell tumours can present as abdominal masses; these are usually ovarian, but may also lead to vaginal bleeding or precocious puberty. Tumour markers - alpha-fetoprotein or beta-HCG - may be raised. Surgery alone can be sufficient to achieve a cure.

Syllabus Mapping

Haematology and Oncology

- Be able to assess, diagnose and make appropriate referral of leukaemias and lymphoproliferative disorders. Be able to assess, diagnose and make appropriate referral of solid tumours

References

1. Maris JM. Recent advances in neuroblastoma [Review]. New England Journal of Medicine 2010; 362: 2202–11.

2. Allen CE, Kelly KM. Bollard CM. Pediatric Lymphomas and Histiocytic Disorders of Childhood [Review]. Pediatric Clinics of North America 2015; 62: 139–165.

3. HaDuong JH, Martin AA, Skapek SX, Mascarenhas L. Sarcomas [Review]. Pediatric Clinics of North America 2015; 62: 179–200.

Further Reading

Hamilton W, Hajioff S, Graham J Schmidt-Hansen M. Suspected cancer (part 1 – children and young adults). BMJ 2015; 350: h3036. doi: 10.1136/bmj.h3036

Davenport KP, Blanco FC, Sandler AD. Pediatric malignancies: Neuroblastoma, Wilm's tumour, hepatoblastoma, rhabdomyosarcoma, and sacroccygeal teratoma [Review]. Surgical Clinics of North America 2012; 92: 745–67.

Irwin MS, Park JR. Neuroblastoma [Review]. Pediatric Clinics of North America 2015; 62: 225–246.

Landier W, Armenian S, Bhatia S. Late effects of childhood cancer and its treatment [Review]. Pediatric Clinics of North America 2015; 62: 275–300.

Chapter 24: A 12 year old boy who presents with bleeding gums
Dr Fiona Hickey, Dr Simone Stokley

(24)

A 12 year old boy presents to the emergency department after having 2 teeth extracted so a brace could be fitted. He has had persistent oozing of blood from the teeth sockets. He does not bruise easily or have prolonged bleeding when he cuts himself. He is otherwise well and has no other significant medical history. He had a tonsillectomy when he was 6 years old and a significant amount of blood was found on the pillow each morning of the week following that operation. He is under the care of a dermatologist for severe eczema.

His father is a plumber who cuts himself on a daily basis but has no problems with prolonged bleeding. His mother is described as "double jointed" and has had 2 Caesarean sections without complications. Her own father had a problem with bleeding after 2 operations. The patient has a brother and a sister who are both well.

Investigations

Blood
Haemoglobin	102 g/l
MCV	77 fl (75–87)
MCH	29 pg (25–37)
MCHC	310 g/l (300–350)
White cell count	8.3 x 10^9/l
Platelets	220 x 10^9/l

Q1. What is the most likely diagnosis?

Select <u>one</u> answer only

A.   Ehlers-Danlos syndrome
B.   Haemophilia A
C.   Haemophilia B
D.   Von Willebrand disease
E.   Wiskott-Aldrich syndrome

A patient known to have severe haemophilia A presents to the emergency department with significant bleeding following dental extraction.

Q2. Which of the following is the most appropriate first-line treatment?

Select <u>one</u> answer only

A.   Cryoprecipitate
B.   Desmopressin
C.   Fresh frozen plasma
D.   Recombinant factor IX
E.   Recombinant factor VIII

Answers and Rationale

Q1.   B: Haemophilia A
Q2.   E: Recombinant factor VIII

Although the mother is described as "double jointed", there is no history of hypermobility in the child to suggest Ehlers-Danlos syndrome. Children with Wiskott-Aldrich syndrome would be expected to have a story of immunodeficiency and thrombocytopaenia. The family history of a bleeding problem for the grandfather but no maternal problems despite major surgery suggests the X-linked disorder haemophilia. The clinical presentation of this case at this age with bleeding after dental extractions is classic for mild haemophilia A (1-3). It is not possible to distinguish haemophilia A and B without formal laboratory testing, but the incidence of A is 1 in 5,000 while B is much less common at 1 in 30,000. Thus, the most likely diagnosis would be haemophilia A

The disorders of clotting or excessive bleeding can be inherited or acquired, and include abnormalities of platelet number or function and clotting factor deficiencies (including von Willebrand disease) (3).

Aspects of the history may give clues to the underlying aetiology. The timing of the first presentation is important, as severe inherited disorders usually present early in life. Occasionally, there may be bleeding from the umbilical stump in the neonatal period that might suggest a factor XIII deficiency or congenital afibrinogenaemia. Thrombocytopaenia can also present at this age, but clotting factor abnormalities are not usually symptomatic in the neonatal period. Excessive bruising becomes more evident when the child starts to mobilise (4).

The type of bleeding experienced by the patient provides important information, as mucocutaneous bleeding (petechiae, purpura or epistaxis) suggests a problem with platelets, von Willebrand disease or a vascular disorder, while bleeding into muscles or joints suggests a clotting factor deficiency. However, those with clotting factor deficiencies can also present with mucocutaneous bleeding after surgery or dental extractions.

Some conditions, such as haemophilia A, haemophilia B and Wiskott-Aldrich, are X-linked, while von Willebrand disease is autosomal dominant and may be evident in the family history.

A bleeding tendency can also be seen with recurrent infections and this would suggest an underlying immune dysfunction, such as those seen in Wiskott-Aldrich or Chediak-Higashi syndromes. More acute systemic symptoms (fever, malaise, and weight loss) in the context of thrombocytopaenia could indicate an underlying malignancy.

An understanding of responses to previous surgeries, dental work or intramuscular immunisations can help distinguish between inherited or acquired clotting problems. Prolonged bleeding or the development of excessive haematomas will raise the prospect of an inherent problem.

Haemophilia A is the result of factor VIII deficiency and haemophilia B is due to factor IX deficiency. Both can present with variable degrees of reduced factor levels, and the severity of the deficiency will guide patient management. Von Willebrand disease is the result of mutations that lead to a reduced production or reduced function of the von Willebrand factor – a protein that is responsible for the adhesion of platelets to the endothelium (3).

The assessment of children who present with concerns regarding excessive bleeding requires an initial full blood count and clotting studies. Any observed thrombocytopaenia requires a review of the blood film to rule out platelet clumps and to assess platelet size and granularity. Even if no platelet clumps are seen, the blood count should always be repeated to confirm the accuracy of the result.

The prothrombin time (PT) assay assesses clotting factors in both extrinsic and common pathways (factors II, V, VII, X and fibrinogen) while the activated partial thromboplastin time (APTT) assesses clotting factors in both the intrinsic and common pathways.

The APPT can be prolonged if inhibitors such as lupus anticoagulant are present. In children, this is usually a post-viral phenomenon that will resolve spontaneously. It can also be prolonged in von Willebrand disease.

Consequently, a prolongation of both the PT and APTT will indicate a deficiency of a factor in the common pathway, but may also be the result of deficiencies of multiple clotting factors. The deficiencies could be acquired, as seen in a vitamin K deficiency or rarely in an inherited combined factor V and VIII deficiency.

Thrombin time (TT) measures the final step of the clotting cascade, when fibrinogen is converted to fibrin by the action of thrombin. An increased TT therefore indicates either decreased levels of fibrinogen or a dysfunctional fibrinogen, although the presence of heparin will also affect the TT and must be considered if an abnormal result is seen.

Von Willebrand disease is the most common inherited bleeding disorder, so specific testing for this condition should be undertaken of there is any history suggestive of a bleeding disorder, even if the APPT is normal (3).

The investigations described so far, however, will not detect disorders of platelet function. It is also important to recognise disseminated intravascular coagulation in the unwell, septic child, as this will lead to a consumption of platelets and clotting factors. Formal testing in such children shows thrombocytopaenia and a low fibrinogen level.

One must always remember that a non-accidental injury may be the cause of abnormal bruising in a child but, at the same time, von Willebrand disease needs to be excluded in a child with excessive bruising.

Syllabus Mapping

Haematology and Oncology

- Be able to assess, diagnose and manage coagulation disorders, hypercoagulable states, purpura and bruising

References and Further Reading

1. Hoffbrand AV, Moss P. Essential Haematology, 7th edition. Blackwell Scientific Publications 2015.

2. Matthews DC et al. Inherited Disorders of Platelet Function. Pediatric Clinics of North America 2013; 60(6): 1476–1488.

3. Kumar R et al. Inherited Abnormalities of Coagulation, Hemophilia, von Willebrand Disease, and Beyond. Pediatric Clinics of North America 2013; 60(6): 1419–1441.

4. Jaffray J et al. Developmental Hemostasis: Clinical Implications From the Fetus to the Adolescent. Pediatric Clinics of North America 2013; 60(6): 1407–1417.

Chapter 25: A 7 year old boy with abdominal pain, wheeze and a rash
Dr Nicola Jay

(25)

A 7 year old asthmatic boy is admitted after becoming unwell at a Christmas party. At the party, he had abdominal pain, vomited, started to wheeze and developed a widespread rash. His mother gave him 4 puffs of his reliever inhaler and called an ambulance.

On arrival in the emergency department, he is given oxygen and receives a 5-mg salbutamol nebuliser and 4 mg of chlorpheniramine syrup. He is pale, with widespread urticaria, and is breathless with a respiratory rate of 28/minute, a heart rate of 102/minute and widespread wheeze on auscultation. His oxygen saturation is 92% in air.

Q1. Which of the following would be the next most appropriate treatment?

Select one answer only

A.   IM adrenaline
B.   IV adrenaline
C.   IV chlorpheniramine
D.   IV hydrocortisone
E.   Nebulised ipratropium bromide
F.   Oral prednisolone
G.   Repeat nebulised salbutamol

Q2. Which of the following blood tests is most likely to be helpful?

Select one answer only

A.   C1 esterase level
B.   C3 and C4 level
C.   Full blood count
D.   Mast cell tryptase
E.   Serum histamine

Answers and Rationale

Q1.   A: IM adrenaline
Q2.   D: Mast cell tryptase

The symptoms of acute abdominal pain with vomiting in association with urticaria and wheeze would suggest an acute allergic reaction. He has failed to respond to oral antihistamines and nebulised bronchodilators. Further nebulised salbutamol, with or without ipratropium bromide, is indicated in a simple asthmatic attack, but is not the primary treatment in a generalised allergic reaction (1, 2).

Acute allergic reactions are classified according to their severity, with any evidence of compromise of the airway, respiratory function or cardiovascular system being grouped as life-threatening. As such, the treatment of choice is adrenaline. Due to the respiratory compromise, intramuscular adrenaline should be used in this case. You may consider nebulised adrenaline for stridor; intravenous adrenaline is only used for cardiac arrest (1, 2). While steroids will also be needed to halt the inflammatory cascade, these are given after the adrenaline.

Current government advice is to avoid whole nuts under the age of 5 due to the risk of choking. Most families avoid all nuts when they could just avoid whole nuts, as this is what young children choke on. However, this advice means that for many children in the UK, the first exposure to nuts is over the age of 5 and is often at a Christmas party. The referral rate for new onset nut allergy has a sharp peak in the New Year (3).

Anaphylaxis is likely when all of the following 3 criteria are met:

• Sudden onset and rapid progression of symptoms

• Life-threatening airway and/or breathing and/or circulation problems

• Skin and/or mucosal changes (flushing, urticaria, angioedema)

The following supports the diagnosis:

• Exposure to a known allergen for the patient

It is important to remember that skin or mucosal changes alone are not a sign of an anaphylactic reaction and that these can be subtle or absent in up to 20% of reactions (some patients can have only a decrease in blood pressure, i.e. a circulation problem). There can also be gastrointestinal symptoms (e.g. vomiting, abdominal pain, incontinence).

The NICE guidance on assessment and management (including referral) of anaphylaxis in adults and children exists. This highlights the importance of clear documentation and the careful assessment that is required to determine whether there are any life-threatening features (airway, breathing or circulation problems).

The NICE guidance recommends that, after a suspected anaphylactic reaction, all adults and young people over the age of 16 should have timed blood samples taken for mast cell tryptase. The first sample should be taken as soon as possible and a second sample should be taken ideally within 1–2 hours of the reaction (but no later than 4 hours).

Blood samples for mast cell tryptase should also be taken in children younger than 16 years who have venom-related, drug-related or idiopathic reactions. In this child, the immediate cause is not known. While you may well suspect nuts as a trigger, this clinical information has not been supplied and so a mast cell tryptase may be very helpful.

Children younger than 16 years who have emergency treatment for suspected anaphylaxis need to be admitted to hospital, as there is a risk of a late (biphasic) reaction. An adrenaline auto-injector prescription and appropriate training in how (and when) to use this are important considerations before discharge. Follow-up with a paediatrician with training in paediatric allergy is important.

While hereditary angioedema is often considered a part of the differential diagnosis in children presenting in this manner, it is an incredibly rare diagnosis. The majority of children will have a family history. If it is considered as a possible diagnosis, then a serum C3 and C4 can be helpful. Normal levels make the diagnosis much less likely, but if there is a very high clinical suspicion, then C1 esterase inhibitor function assays are required to exclude the diagnosis.

Syllabus Mapping

Emergency Medicine (including accidents and poisoning)

- Be able to assess, diagnose and manage children presenting with anaphylaxis including acute life threatening upper airways obstruction

Infection, Immunology, Allergy

- Be able to assess, diagnose and manage allergies

References

1. Huang F, Chawla K, Jarvinen KM, Nowak-Weegrzyn. Anaphylaxis in a New York City pediatric emergency department: Triggers, treatment and outcomes. *JACI* 2011,129: 162–168.

2. RCPCH Care Pathway for Anaphylaxis 2012: 1–11. www.rcpch.ac.uk.

3. Turner PJ, Gowland MH, Sharma V et al. Increase in anaphylaxis-related hospitalisations but no increase in fatalities: An analysis of United Kingdom national anaphylaxis data, 2002–2012. *JACI* 2015; 135: 956–963.

Further Reading

NICE guidelines (CG134). Anaphylaxis: Assessment and referral after emergency treatment. https://www.nice.org.uk/guidance/cg134.

Chapter 26: A 5 year old girl with wrist pain
Dr Samundeeswari Deepak, Dr Kishore Warrier

(26)

A 5 year old girl is seen in a general paediatric clinic with a 6 week history of episodic pain and stiffness affecting her wrists, ankles and right knee. In her detailed history, she had a swollen and painful right knee a year ago that was thought to be the result of trauma, and this settled down quickly with analgesia and rest. Since then, she has suffered with pain and swelling in different joints. There are no other symptoms. Her father was a professional footballer who had surgery to his left knee and her mother had eczema. On examination, she looks well but is slightly pale. Her temperature is 37.6°C. There are no obvious dermatological abnormalities. Examination of her joints shows obvious swelling without erythema of her right knee and left wrist. There is a limitation of movement of neck flexion, wrists, right knee and left ankle. Her spine demonstrates the limitation of flexion. The rest of the examination is normal.

Investigations

Blood

Haemoglobin	98 g/l
MCV	72 fl (75–87)
MCH	23 pg (25–37)
MCHC	290 g/l (300–350)
White cell count	14.5 x 10^9/l
Platelets	460 x 10^9/l
ESR	63 mm/hr
CRP	20 mg/l
Rheumatoid factor	Negative
ANA	Negative

Q1. What is the likely diagnosis?

Select <u>one</u> answer only

A.   Ankylosing spondylitis
B.   Lyme disease
C.   Polyarticular juvenile arthritis
D.   Systemic juvenile arthritis
E.   Systemic lupus erythematosus

Q2. Which is the next most important investigation?

Select <u>one</u> answer only

A.   Borrelia burgdorferi titres
B.   Echocardiography
C.   ECG
D.   Lung function testing
E.   Plain x-ray of affected joints
F.   Slit lamp examination

Answer and Rationale

Q1. **C: Polyarticular juvenile arthritis**
Q2. **F: Slit lamp examination**

This young girl presents with 5 swollen joints developing over a 6-week period. She has limitation of movement in multiple joints. The absence of obvious dermatological findings makes Lyme disease, systemic lupus erythematosus and systemic juvenile arthritis unlikely. A microcytic and hypochromic anaemia and raised ESR support the diagnosis of polyarticular juvenile arthritis.

Uveitis in juvenile idiopathic arthritis (JIA) is most often asymptomatic and needs regular screening under a slit lamp for early diagnosis and treatment.

JIA is essentially a clinical diagnosis and one of exclusion with a wide range of differential diagnoses. It is the most common chronic rheumatological disease in children (1).

JIA is defined as joint inflammation in those under the age of 16 years, and persisting for at least 6 weeks. Other potential cause must be excluded. Classically, a joint affected by arthritis is swollen and painful with some restriction of movement, although the history of pain is often absent in the younger child. Parents may describe a child as refusing to stand or having a limp first thing in the morning, but as running about normally later in the day. It may also be an explanation for delay in the development of motor skills.

The pathogenesis and aetiology of JIA are unclear, although interactions between genetic factors, immune mechanisms and environmental exposures are all thought to contribute. T lymphocytes have a central role in the inflammatory response and they release pro-inflammatory cytokines such as TNF-α, IL-1 and IL-6. The chronic inflammation of synovium is characterised by B-lymphocyte infiltration and expansion. Rheumatoid factor assays detect IgM antibodies directed against the Fc portion of IgG molecules, whereas antinuclear antibodies (ANA) usually target specific antigens in the cell nuclei (2).

Up to 7 subsets of JIA are recognised in international classifications, but there are 3 types that are commonly seen and each has a differing clinical course (3).

Oligoarticular JIA, present in 50% of patients, is often seen in early childhood and usually affects the large joints (knees, ankles and wrists), most commonly in girls. Up to 4 joints may be involved, although half may only have a monoarthritis. Uveitis occurs in up to 30% of patients and ANA is positive in 50–70%.

Polyarticular JIA, again, is more common in girls and affects 5 or more joints in a symmetrical manner. Children can either be positive (RF+) or negative (RF-) for rheumatoid factor. Rheumatoid factor negative polyarticular JIA is the most common (25% of all patients), and these patients have a risk of developing uveitis particularly if they are ANA positive. Those who are rheumatoid factor positive can progress to the classical rheumatoid arthritis seen in adulthood with the risk of severe erosive arthropathy.

Children presenting with systemic JIA are often between 4–7 years and account for around 10% of all patients. They frequently have a salmon-pink, macular, intermittent rash along with lymphadenopathy and hepatosplenomegaly. The arthritis, which is usually symmetrical and affects several joints, may not develop for some weeks or months after the appearance of the rash. The clinical picture can simulate infection or malignancy.

Psoriatic arthritis is often asymmetrical and may affect finger joints, giving dactylitis. The arthritis may develop before the psoriasis but a positive family history will suggest the likely aetiological mechanism.

Enthesitis-related arthritis describes an inflammatory process at the site of muscle insertion, leading to pain and erythema. Lower limb joints are usually affected, particularly the ankle. The young person is at risk of uveitis and inflammatory bowel disease, and investigations may identify a personal or family history of HLA-B27 positivity.

The juvenile arthritides can mimic many other conditions and will often require a structured approach to investigation. Trauma, localised and systemic infection and malignancy may all be included in an early differential diagnosis, and plain x-rays, which are normal in early JIA, can be useful to exclude these. MRI will delineate any bony changes, joint damage and the extent of synovitis.

The goal of management is to provide early treatment and thus prevent long-term joint and eye damage.

Medical treatment will involve the use of non-steroidal anti-inflammatory drugs such as ibuprofen in the first instance. Thereafter, the approach is to arrest the inflammatory process with corticosteroids (intra-articular or systemic) and to maintain this position with disease-modifying anti-rheumatic drugs (DMARDs). Oral or subcutaneous methotrexate given each week is used in this way. An inadequate response to methotrexate requires an escalation to biological cytokine modulators (etanercept, infliximab or adalimumab), which inhibit the effects of TNF. Many of these agents are also used for the treatment of uveitis that does not respond to topical steroid therapy.

Surgical interventions such as joint replacement or synovectomy are rarely required now due to advances in medical management.

The long-term outlook for children and young people who are diagnosed with JIA is very good, as the disease is often self-limiting. About 60% of patients can be expected to reach adulthood with no active synovitis or functional limitation. The disease, however, can be unpredictable and exacerbations can occur.

Syllabus Mapping

Musculoskeletal

- Be able to assess, diagnose and manage musculoskeletal disorders including those with systemic manifestations, acute and chronic arthritis and know when to refer

References

1. Foster H, Brogan PA (eds). Juvenile Idiopathic arthritis. In: Oxford Handbook of Paediatric Rheumatology. Oxford University Press 2012.

2. Mehta, J. Laboratory Testing in Pediatric Rheumatology. Pediatric Clinics of North America 2012; 59(2): 263-284.

3. Petty RE, Southwood TR, Manners P et al. International League of Associations for Rheumatology classification of juvenile idiopathic arthritis: Second revision. J Rheumatol 2004; 31(2): 390-2.

Further Reading

Berard, R. Approach to the Child with Joint Inflammation. Pediatric Clinics of North America 2012; 59(2): 245-262.

Gowdie, PJ et al. Juvenile Idiopathic Arthritis. Pediatric Clinics of North America 2012; 59(2): 301-327.

Cassidy JT, Petty RE. Chronic arthritis in childhood. In: Cassidy JT, Petty RE, Laxer RM, Lindsley CB (eds). Textbook of Pediatric Rheumatology, 5th edition. Elsevier Saunders: Philadelphia, 2005.

Chapter 27: A newborn baby with generalised oedema
Dr Helen Chitty, Dr Mithilesh Lal

(27)

A male infant born at 34 weeks of gestation is noted to be oedematous and pale, with poor respiratory effort and shallow breathing soon after birth. His birthweight is 2.9 kg. He is admitted to the neonatal unit and is commenced on nasal CPAP of 5 cm (H_2O) and supplemental oxygen.

Further examination reveals a heart rate of 170/minute, respiratory rate of 60/minute, and a slightly distended abdomen with generalised oedema. His mother moved to the UK recently, and a late antenatal booking blood test confirms her blood group as O Rh negative. She has a 3 year old daughter who was born at 39 weeks of gestation in Egypt, and was treated with phototherapy for jaundice.

A chest x-ray taken at about 4 hours of age shows features of poor aeration and obliteration of costophrenic angles on both sides.

Q1. Which of the following investigations would give the most definite confirmation that the baby has got alloimmune haemolytic disease?

Select <u>one</u> answer only

A.	Blood group and rhesus typing
B.	Direct antiglobulin test
C.	Full blood count and peripheral blood film
D.	Reticulocyte count
E.	Serum bilirubin level

The infant's initial blood tests on admission are reported at 4 hours of age and show:

Haemoglobin	87g/l
Total bilirubin	100 µmol/l
Direct antiglobulin test	positive
Blood group	O Rhesus positive

Intensive phototherapy treatment is commenced.

Q2. What is the most important management indicated in addition to phototherapy?

Select <u>one</u> answer only

A.	Exchange transfusion
B.	Hearing screen
C.	IVIG
D.	Packed cell blood transfusion
E.	Recheck the serum bilirubin level in 6 hours

Answers and Rationale

Q1. **B: Direct antiglobulin test**
Q2. **A: Exchange transfusion**

Rhesus incompatibility between mother and fetus still remains one of the causes of haemolytic disease of the newborn (HDN). Rhesus HDN (Rh HDN) occurs when the red blood cells of a rhesus antigen-negative mother are exposed to the red blood cells of a rhesus antigen-positive fetus (1). If this occurs, the mother produces IgG antibodies that cross the placenta and bind to the rhesus antigens on the fetal red blood cells.

The process by which mothers are initially exposed to fetal rhesus antigens is known as 'sensitisation' or 'alloimmunisation' (also described as isoimmunisation). This first exposure may not cause any clinical effects in the fetus or newborn infant, but exposure to fetal rhesus antigens in subsequent pregnancies will lead to the production of maternal IgG antibodies that cross the placenta and bind to fetal rhesus antigens. This leads to haemolysis of red blood cells that can occur antenatally and can continue postnatally.

There are several different rhesus antigens. Rhesus D antigens were the most common cause of Rh HDN until the introduction of intramuscular IgG anti-D injections that are administered to rhesus D antigen-negative women during or after pregnancy. The aim of these injections is to prevent maternal sensitisation (see below). Other rhesus antigens occur less commonly but are now increasingly the cause of Rh HDN. These antigens include Rh C and Rh c antigens, Rh C^W antigens, and Rh E and Rh e antigens.

Alloimmunisation due to other red blood cell antigens (see the box below) has become more common since the widespread use of anti-D immunoglobulin for Rh HDN (2). Apart from Rh and ABO antigens, the Kell antigen is the most immunogenic. There are 25 different Kell antigens encoded on chromosome 7. Pathophysiology of Kell alloimmunisation differs from that of ABO and Rh disease in that Kell IgG antibody can cause macrophage-mediated destruction of erythroid precursors in the fetal liver, leading to severe anaemia. Kell haemolytic disease is still rare, as 91% of the population is Kell negative and only 5% of the population form antibodies following a blood transfusion.

> Atypical antibodies associated with HDN include Kell, Duffy, Kidd, MNSs, MSS, Diego, P, En, Co, Heibel, radin, Wright, and Zd.

HDN can present in different ways. The infant may appear well at delivery but may quickly become jaundiced. HDN can lead to severe hyperbilirubinaemia and kernicterus, if left untreated. Jaundice can be managed with phototherapy, regular clinical reviews of the infant and the monitoring of the serum bilirubin and haemoglobin levels. Anaemia can be mild, moderate or severe. If it occurs before birth, it can lead to cardiac impairment and subsequent oedema. Haemolysis can continue for several weeks after birth; thus, an infant who is not initially anaemic may slowly become severely anaemic over the first few weeks of life.

Assessment and monitoring of fetal anaemia previously required invasive tests such as cordocentesis for fetal blood sampling and amniocentesis for optical density of bilirubin in the amniotic fluid. This has now been replaced by Doppler flow studies for peak velocity in the middle cerebral artery; a peak systolic velocity of >1.5 shows a good correlation with fetal anaemia.

Only the direct antiglobulin test is specific for alloimmune haemolytic disease. However, infants of mothers who have received anti-D injections may have weakly positive direct antiglobulin tests even in the absence of alloimmunisation. Risk of alloimmune sensitisation depends on the volume of fetomaternal haemorrhage, and a minimum of 0.25 ml is thought to be needed. The risk of fetomaternal bleeding increases gradually from the first to the third trimester, and is the maximum at delivery (17%). Simultaneous ABO incompatibility between mother and the fetus in pregnancies with Rh sensitisation tends to reduce sensitisation. Quantifiable fetomaternal bleeding appears to occur in over 75% of all pregnancies.

Apart from phototherapy, regular monitoring of blood tests and good supportive care, another important aspect of the management of severe HDN is erythrocyte replacement. This is not considered in all cases, but is considered in severe cases of haemolysis. A severely anaemic fetus can be transfused before birth (in utero transfusion) to prevent the detrimental effects of anaemia.

After birth, a newborn infant may receive an exchange transfusion in which the infant's blood is removed in small aliquots and replaced by donor blood. The aim of the exchange transfusion is to replace the infant's red blood cells (which contain the antigen-antibody complex causing the ongoing haemolysis), remove the maternal red blood cells in the infant's circulation, and remove the excess serum bilirubin. An infant may require more than 1 exchange transfusion. Slow, chronic anaemia occurring during the first few weeks of life may eventually require a 'top-up' blood transfusion.

High-dose IVIG has been shown to be effective in reducing the bilirubin levels, and reduces the need for exchange transfusion in rhesus or ABO immune haemolytic disease. It is used as an adjunct to intensive phototherapy if the serum bilirubin continues to increase by >8.5 µmol/l/hour (3). The mechanism of action of IVIG is the non-specific blockade of IgG antibody receptors (known as Fc receptors). Maternal IVIG administration also reduces fetal haemolysis.

Syllabus Mapping

Neonatology

- Be able to initiate and interpret diagnostic tests and plan initial management of the conditions that cause neonatal jaundice

Haematology and Oncology

- Understand the risks, benefits and precautions involved in blood transfusion

References and Further Reading

1. Waldron PE and Cashore WJ. Hemolytic disease of the fetus and newborn. In: de Alarcón P and Werner E (eds). Neonatal Hematology. 1st edition. Cambridge University Press: Cambridge, 2005: 91–131.

2. Diab Y and Luchtman-Jones L. The blood and haematopoietic system. Part 1: Hematologic and oncologic problems in the fetus and neonate. In: Martin RJ, Fanaroff AA, Walsh MC (eds). Fanaroff and Martin's Neonatal-Perinatal Medicine: Diseases of the Fetus and Infant, 10th edition. Elsevier Saunders, 2015: 1294–1343.

3. National Institute for Health and Clinical Excellence: Clinical Guidance on Neonatal Jaundice. www.nice.org.uk/CG98.

Chapter 28: An 11 month old girl with fever and abdominal pain
Dr Alison Davies, Dr Martin Hewitt

(28)

An 11 month old girl is admitted to the paediatric ward with a 2 day history of fever and abdominal pain. Past history includes episodic temperatures without identified focus.

The examination shows her to be withdrawn, fractious and flushed. Her temperature is 38.5°C and her heart rate is 120/minute. Blood pressure is 91/63 mmHg. An examination of ears, throat and chest shows no abnormalities. An examination of the abdomen shows it to be soft without guarding but some tenderness in the suprapubic area and tenderness in the loin area. There are no masses and her bowel sounds are normal. A bag urine is obtained and urine dipstick is positive for nitrites and leukocytes. The sample is sent for culture and sensitivities.

Q1. What would be your next most appropriate step in the management of this child?

Select <u>one</u> answer only

A.   Obtain a clean catch urine and then start IV antibiotics
B.   Obtain a clean catch urine and then start oral antibiotics
C.   Obtain a clean catch urine but await culture results before starting antibiotics
D.   Obtain a second urine sample by suprapubic aspiration, after which start IV antibiotics
E.   Obtain a second urine sample by suprapubic aspiration, after which start oral antibiotics

The culture result from the second urine sample shows an isolated growth of Klebsiella.

Q2. Which of the following imaging schedules is appropriate?

Select <u>one</u> answer only

A.   No imaging in the acute period but renal tract ultrasound only within 6 weeks
B.   No imaging is necessary
C.   Renal tract ultrasound and MCUG within 6 weeks
D.   Renal tract ultrasound scan during the acute infection; if normal, no further investigations
E.   Renal tract ultrasound scan during the acute infection with DMSA scan 6 months post-acute infection

Answers and Rationale

Q1.   **E: Obtain a second urine sample by suprapubic aspiration, after which start oral antibiotics**
Q2.   **E: Renal tract ultrasound scan during the acute infection with DMSA scan 6 months post-acute infection**

In this question, an 11 month old girl has an <u>atypical</u> (infection with a non-*E. coli* organism) upper UTI (temperature >38°C and bacteriuria with Klebsiella). She is over 6 months of age and could therefore be treated with a 10-day course of oral antibiotics. Obtaining a second urine sample by suprapubic aspiration will allow a confident interpretation of the clinical picture and direct further investigations.

A renal tract ultrasound during the acute infection is required to exclude structural abnormalities and a delayed DMSA scan at 4–6 months to exclude renal scarring.

The current UK guidelines are produced by NICE (1). The need to confirm the diagnosis of UTI is important to identify children at risk of renal tract abnormalities and future UTIs. It also avoids potentially unnecessary invasive investigations.

Infants and children presenting with an unexplained fever or symptoms of a UTI should have a urine sample tested for infection. In infants younger than 3 months of age, signs and symptoms could include fever, vomiting, lethargy, irritability and poor feeding and, less commonly, jaundice, haematuria and abdominal pain. In older children, additional, more specific features may also be present, including loin tenderness, dysuria, increased frequency and cloudy or offensive urine (2).

A bag urine sample is inappropriate for bacteriological use; a clean catch urine sample is preferable and should be sent for microscopy and culture. In children 3 years and older, dipstick testing for leukocyte esterase and nitrites is diagnostically as useful as a microscopy and can safely be used to diagnose a UTI, but a sample should also be sent for culture to obtain the organism and sensitivities.

If nitrites are positive on the dipstick, antibiotic treatment should be started for a suspected UTI. If only leukocytes are present, a repeat urine sample should be sent for microscopy and culture and antibiotics should only be started if there is good clinical evidence for a UTI.

Infants and children who have loin pain or tenderness and bacteriuria (or who have a fever of over 38°C along with a bacteriuria) should be considered to have acute pyelonephritis or upper UTI. A UTI that does not fit these criteria should be regarded as a lower UTI.

Infants less than 3 months of age should be treated for a suspected UTI with parenteral antibiotics irrespective of which site (upper or lower) is considered. Those older than 3 months with an upper UTI (acute pyelonephritis) can be treated with oral antibiotics for 7–10 days, while those with a lower UTI should be treated with oral antibiotics for 3 days. Local guidelines should be consulted to determine the most appropriate antibiotic to be used. All children should be reviewed at 48 hours, with the result of the culture, to assess response to treatment and ensure the organism is sensitive to the prescribed antibiotic.

The majority of children with UTI have normal renal tracts and are not at risk of any long-term sequelae. Risk factors for renal tract abnormalities include young age, recurrent UTI and atypical UTI. Renal parenchymal defects can be seen in these groups and, if bilateral, are associated with hypertension, proteinuria and complications in pregnancy. Rarely can they progress to established renal failure.

A recurrent UTI is defined as more than 1 upper UTI (pyelonephritis) or more than 2 lower UTIs. Infants and children with recurrent UTIs require further investigations and should therefore be considered for antibiotic prophylaxis.

An atypical UTI should be considered if the child was seriously ill, had a palpable bladder, had a raised creatinine, had a failed response to appropriate antibiotics, or had an infection with non-*E. coli* organisms.

Infants and children with an atypical UTI should have an ultrasound of the urinary tract during the acute infection to identify structural abnormalities of the urinary tract, such as obstruction.

Infants under the age of 6 months with recurrent or atypical UTIs should have an ultrasound during the acute phase. They also need a DMSA scan in the next 4–6 months to look for evidence of renal scarring and an MCUG to exclude vesico-ureteric reflux (VUR) or posterior urethral valves (PUV) (3). A child in this age group with a first infection and who responds promptly to antibiotics should have a delayed renal ultrasound at 6 weeks to exclude structural abnormalities.

Those children between 6 months and 3 years of age with either atypical or recurrent UTIs also need a DMSA scan in the next 4–6 months following the acute infection to identify possible renal scarring. Those in this age group who do not have an atypical UTI and who respond promptly within the first 48 hours to antibiotics do not need any further investigations.

Children over 3 years of age who have recurrent infections are advised to have a DMSA scan to identify renal scarring.

An MCUG is not required in those over 6 months, as older children are much less likely to have undiagnosed VUR or PUV and it is the most invasive of investigations.

Syllabus Mapping

Nephro-urology

- Be able to assess, diagnose and manage nephro-urological disorders, including those with systemic manifestations and make appropriate referral

- Be able to assess, diagnose and manage urinary tract infection with appropriate referral

References

1. NICE guideline (CG54). Urinary tract infection in under 16s: Diagnosis and management August 2007. https://www.nice.org.uk/guidance/cg54

2. Downs SM. Technical Report: Urinary Tract Infections in Febrile Infants and Young Children. Pediatrics 1999; 103(4). http://www.pediatrics.org/cgi/content/full/103/4/e54.

3. Tullus K. Vesicoureteric reflux in children. Lancet 2015; 385: 371–9.

Further Reading

Koyle MA, Shifrin D. Issues in febrile urinary tract infection management . Pediatric Clinics of North America 2012; 59(4): 909–22.

Montini G, Tullus K, Hewitt I. Febrile urinary tract infections in children. NEJM 2011; 365(3): 239-50.

Chapter 29: A 3 year old boy admitted with lethargy
Dr Andrew Maxted, Dr Andrew Lunn

(29)

A 3 year old boy is admitted to hospital with a week-long history of progressive lethargy and sleepiness. He is drinking slightly more than usual but his appetite has reduced over this time period. There are no other specific symptoms and, in particular, no indication of headaches or visual disturbances. His parents and one sibling are well and there are no known illnesses in the family. He is not taking any regular medications apart from the occasional paracetamol.

On examination, he is drowsy but rousable and his Glasgow Coma Scale score is recorded as 10. His eyes are 'slightly sunken'. His heart rate is 150/minute and his blood pressure is 70/45 mmHg. Heart sounds are normal. Respiration rate is 34/minute, there is no recession and breath sounds are normal. No abnormalities are found on examination of the abdomen and neurological systems – fundi are normal.

Investigations

Blood

Sodium	166 mmol/l
Potassium	5.3 mmol/l
Bicarbonate	28 mmol/l
Urea	10.1 mmol/l
Creatinine	144 µmol/l
Glucose	6.1 mmol/l

Urine

Normal dipstick
Osmolality (first morning) – 150 mosm/kg

Q1. What is the most likely cause of his electrolyte abnormalities?

Select <u>one</u> answer only

A. Nephrogenic diabetes insipidus (NDI)
B. Primary hyperaldosteronism
C. Rotavirus causing vomiting
D. Salt poisoning
E. Syndrome of inappropriate antidiuretic hormone (SIADH)

Q2. What is the most appropriate fluid regime to provide at this time?

Select <u>one</u> answer only

A. IV fluids at maintenance rate with 0.18% saline/5% dextrose
B. IV fluids at maintenance rate plus 10% with 0.9% saline
C. IV fluids at maintenance rate plus 10% with 0.18% saline/5% dextrose
D. Oral fluids at maintenance rate plus 10% with 0.45% saline/5% dextrose
E. Oral fluids at maintenance rate plus 10% without saline

Answers and Rationale

Q1. **A: Nephrogenic diabetes insipidus (NDI)**
Q2. **E: Oral fluids at maintenance rate plus 10% without saline**

The history indicates a recent onset of lethargy without any indications of a neural cause. The investigations show hypernatraemia with a normal potassium level and low urine osmolality, and there is evidence of dehydration. Primary hyperaldosteronism leads to sodium retention and potassium loss and SIADH causes hyponatraemia due to inappropriate retention of water without a change in the sodium balance. Neither would fit the clinical picture in this case. NDI, dehydration and salt poisoning produce hypernatraemia with normal potassium. The hypernatraemic dehydration seen as a result of excessive water loss would be associated with a high urine osmolality, as the kidneys attempt to conserve water. Salt poisoning would be associated with a high urine osmolality as the body attempts to excrete sodium, and with clinical features of water retention (1).

The picture of hypernatraemia in the face of low urine osmolality is consistent with NDI, in which the kidneys continue to excrete water despite dehydration. NDI may be congenital or acquired. Congenital NDI usually presents in the first year of life, but 13% of patients present later than 30 months of age. Acquired NDI is generally the result of an acute severe kidney injury.

When correcting hypernatraemic dehydration, the use of enteral fluids in a patient who can tolerate them capitalises on the normal homeostatic mechanism. Using intravenous fluids may force an obligatory further excretion of water to accommodate any infused sodium.

Sodium homeostasis is linked with water and plasma volume. The kidneys do not directly measure sodium levels, but use a combination of the renin-angiotensin-aldosterone axis and anti-diuretic hormone (ADH) to control both sodium reabsorption (and hence water absorption due to osmotic pressure) and water reabsorption directly. Disorders of sodium levels are usually (but not always) caused by abnormalities in plasma tonicity – i.e. the 'effective' osmolality of plasma. It is this 'effective' osmolality that is sensed by cellular osmoreceptors and determines the distribution of water. Normal plasma osmolality is 275 to 290 mosmol/kg and is produced mainly by sodium solutes. Sodium is largely an extracellular electrolyte and, in hypernatraemia, this increased tonicity pulls water out of the cells and results in a decrease in intracellular volume.

Normal homeostasis of sodium is largely driven by the osmotic pressure and blood pressure supplying the kidney. In response to a low blood pressure or low osmolality, the juxtaglomerular cells release renin, which leads to the release of angiotensin 2.

Angiotensin 2 increases peripheral vasoconstriction, ADH release from the anterior pituitary, aldosterone release from the adrenal glands, and sodium, bicarbonate absorption and water from the proximal tubules of the kidney.

Aldosterone acts upon the distal convoluted tubule to increase reabsorption of sodium ions (and thereby water) at the expense of potassium and hydrogen ions. This results in hypokalaemia and the production of acidic urine. ADH acts upon the distal convoluted tubules and the collecting duct system to increase water reabsorption.

Hypernatraemia is defined as a sodium level that is greater than 145 mmol/l, and the causes can be classified as those in which body water volume is reduced (from inappropriate loss or insufficient intake) or those in which the body sodium intake is excessive. The former are associated with evidence of dehydration and weight loss, while the latter usually involve volume expansion and thus weight gain. Prompt treatment is required but it is important to obtain appropriate blood and urine samples, as laboratory values can change quickly.

Hypernatraemic dehydration is sometimes seen in breastfed babies as a result of reduced fluid intake while breastfeeding is being established. These babies are dehydrated, have lost weight, have an increased capillary refill time and often have very high sodium levels. Younger children, similarly, are at risk of hypernatraemic dehydration as a result of inadequate fluid intake (2).

Assessment of urinary sodium can help in the management of fluids in those patients with abnormalities of serum sodium. Fractional excretion of sodium (FENa) measures the excreted (urinary) sodium and expresses this as a percentage of filtered sodium. Values of the FENa under 1% suggest a pre-renal problem, as almost all of the filtered sodium is being reabsorbed, while values of FENa above 2% indicate significant renal injury.

Concentrated urine (urine osmolality greater than plasma osmolality) and minimal urine sodium indicate that the kidneys are attempting to reabsorb sodium and water in response to the low plasma volume. This is usually found in extra-renal fluid loss, such as from the GI tract (diarrhoea and vomiting) or inadequate intake, including an impaired thirst mechanism.

Dilute urine (plasma osmolality greater than urine osmolality) and minimal urine sodium demonstrates that the kidneys are inappropriately releasing dilute urine in the presence of reduced plasma volume. The recognised cause is diabetes insipidus (DI). A water deprivation test is required to confirm the diagnosis.

The production of dilute urine with excessive amounts of sodium in the urine indicates that the kidneys are inappropriately losing sodium. This would be seen following diuretic administration, in osmotic diuresis secondary to glycosuria, and a post-obstructive diuresis.

If the patient has a normal circulating volume and is hypernatraemic but is found to have high urinary sodium levels (urine osmolality greater than plasma osmolality), then the kidneys are trying to excrete sodium and water in response to a high sodium intake (iatrogenic, accidental or salt poisoning).

An accurate assessment of the fluid status of the patient who is hypernatraemic will guide further investigations and management. Those who are dehydrated and shocked will require resuscitation with intravenous 0.9% saline and subsequent reassessment. Children who are dehydrated but not shocked will benefit from a slow correction – preferably using fluids administered enterally. Rapid correction of hypernatraemia can cause cerebral osmotic shifts and significant cerebral injury. Those who are not dehydrated should again have a slow correction of the fluid deficit by enteral water intake that exceeds the sodium intake.

Administered sodium in replaced fluids should be calculated and balanced with the requirements of the child. Normal saline (0.9%) contains 154 mmol/l, and 1500 ml of this fluid will provide 231 mmol of sodium. A 5 year old child who weighs 20kg would therefore receive over 11 mmol/kg per day, which is many times the normal daily requirements.

Syllabus Mapping

Nephro-urology

*   Be able to assess, diagnose and manage nephro-urological disorders, including those with systemic manifestations and make appropriate referral

References

1. Royal College of Paediatrics and Child Health. The differential diagnosis of hypernatraemia in children, with particular reference to salt poisoning, published Sep 2009.

2. Modi N. Avoiding hypernatraemic dehydration in healthy term infants. Archives of Disease in Childhood 2009; 92(6): 474–5.

Further Reading

Rees L, Brogan PA, Bockenhauer D, Webb JA. Paediatric Nephrology (Oxford Specialist Handbooks in Paediatrics) Oxford University Press, 2012.

Robroch AH, van Heerde M, Markhorst DG. Should isotonic infusion solutions routinely be used in hospitalised paediatric patients? Archives of Disease in Childhood 2011; 96(6): 608–10.

Conley SB. Hypernatremia. Pediatric Clinics of North America 1990; 37(2): 365–72.

Chapter 30: A child with a troublesome wheeze
Dr Rob Primhak, Dr Will Carroll

(30)

A 6 year old boy is referred to the clinic due to a recurrent cough and wheeze for the past 2 years. These are present most days but are worse with colds. His GP prescribed 2 puffs of a salbutamol inhaler through a large-volume spacer, which relieves the symptoms, but he needs to use it once or twice almost every day and is coughing a lot at night. He was then started on beclometasone dipropionate in the form of clenil modulite 200 µg twice a day through a spacer. His technique appears appropriate and his GP feels that the family is adhering to treatment. Both parents say they smoke, but only outside the house.

On examination, his height and weight are on the 75th centile. There is no cyanosis or clubbing, but he has a Harrison's sulcus, and a mildly increased thoracic anteroposterior diameter. You hear occasional scattered wheezes on auscultation. His spirometry demonstrates a forced expiratory volume in 1 second of 83% of predicted and a forced vital capacity of 96%. His fractional exhaled nitric oxide (FeNO) is 56 parts per billion.

Q1. What is the most appropriate management?

Select <u>one</u> answer only

A.   Add inhaled salmeterol 50 µg twice a day
B.   Add oral montelukast 5 mg daily
C.   Change the preventer to inhaled budesonide 200 µg twice a day via dry powder inhaler
D.   Change the preventer to inhaled fluticasone propionate 125 µg twice a day
E.   Increase clenil modulite to 400 µg twice a day

He returns for review 3 months later. His symptoms have not improved and his lung function and FeNO measurement remain unchanged.

Q2. What is the most likely reason for the apparent failure of the therapy?

Select <u>one</u> answer only

A.   He is not taking his preventer inhaler regularly
B.   He has inhaled a foreign body
C.   He has steroid-resistant asthma
D.   His inhaler technique is poor at home
E.   His parents are smokers

Answer and Rationale

Q1. **A: Add inhaled salmeterol 50 μg twice a day**
Q2. **A: He is not taking his preventer inhaler regularly**

The two main patterns of wheezing at this age are wheezing solely with colds (viral episodic wheeze) and wheezing to more than 1 trigger, which can be regarded as asthma (1). It should be noted, however, that colds are also the most common trigger of asthma attacks in children with multi-trigger wheeze. Viral episodic wheeze may respond to a leukotriene receptor antagonist, such as montelukast, either for short courses at the onset of the cold or as ongoing therapy. There is less evidence to support the use of inhaled steroids in this type of wheeze. In contrast, inhaled steroids are the first-line preventive therapy for children with asthma (multi-trigger wheeze).

In clinical practice, the first question to ask in this situation is whether there is sufficient evidence to make a diagnosis of asthma. Is the noise that is reported as wheeze a genuine wheeze? Are there symptoms that make asthma less likely, such as a persistent wet cough, onset from birth, other noises such as stridor, associated chronic ENT disease or other infections? Are there atypical signs, such as clubbing, localised crackles, or faltering growth (2). In this case, the wheeze is present on examination, it is said to improve with salbutamol, and there are no features suggesting other diagnoses, although the presence of a chest deformity suggests a sustained period of under-treatment.

The examiners have made it easier still, as the only options available in question 1 are increases in asthma treatment. They have also given you a set of spirometry readings, where the forced expiratory volume is lower (as a percentage predicted) than the forced vital capacity. To seal the diagnosis, there is an elevated fractional FeNO.

We are now left with the question of what pharmacological step is best when a child of 5 does not respond adequately to an initial dose of inhaled steroids. The British Thoracic Society/SIGN guidelines (1) recommend that, under the age of 5, the next step is the addition of montelukast. In children aged 5 or older, the recommended next step is the addition of a long-acting beta-agonist (LABA) such as salmeterol. The normal recommended starting dose of an inhaled steroid in a child of this age is 100–200 micrograms daily of beclometasone or equivalent, so this child is already on a higher than average dose, and it would not be appropriate to increase the dose further at this point without trying additional therapies. Whenever possible, LABA should be given in combination with inhaled steroids, as monotherapy with LABA increases the risk of severe asthma exacerbation and death.

There is no evidence that one steroid is superior to another in equipotent dosage, so there is little point in changing to a different steroid at this stage, unless there is a strong patient preference for a particular device. Budesonide and beclometasone are roughly equipotent, and fluticasone has about twice the potency of the other two. There are differences in oral bioavailability, with fluticasone having almost none (approximately 0.5%), and budesonide having less than beclometasone, but this is of little relevance if they are given by a large-volume spacer that minimises oropharyngeal deposition.

The use of dry powder devices is not recommended for children under 7 years in any type of case, and therefore option C is incorrect.

The other management option that might be considered in this case would be a short course of oral steroids while commencing the additional treatment. In patients with poorly controlled asthma, there may be a degree of steroid resistance; this can be improved by bringing the asthma under control. This option was not offered in the answers to avoid confusion.

While a change in treatment is often effective, a significant proportion of children who return to the clinic report that their symptoms have not improved. Understanding why a child has not improved is essential, but, in this case and in clinical practice, there is often significant guesswork involved. In clinical practice, more than one factor may be playing a part in an individual child's case.

Is he being given the therapy effectively?

The history suggests that he is, although objective measures of adherence suggest that doctors are not good at identifying patients with poor adherence. Are there extraneous factors in the home that might worsen his symptoms, such as pets or smokers? The house dust mite is fairly ubiquitous in British homes, and there is no evidence that attempts to reduce exposure have a significant impact on asthma control. Passive smoking is certainly a factor that can worsen asthma control and the parents' claim that they smoke only outside of the house should be taken with a pinch of salt, but it is less likely to be responsible for such a poor response to treatment.

Obviously, advice and support to quit should be offered routinely to smoking parents of any child with respiratory symptoms. Psychological factors may also need to be explored, especially in an older child with asthma that is difficult to control.

In the present case, the information given is limited, but data from randomised controlled trials including children of this age have shown that a very large proportion adhere poorly to regular treatment (3). This can be improved significantly with the use of reminders (mean adherence was 30% in the group without a reminder, and 84% in the reminder group).

In some instances, a candid discussion with the parents and child will reveal that the main issue has been one of intentional or unintentional non-adherence. In this situation, it may be appropriate to keep the treatment unchanged. The fractional excretion of nitric oxide in this child is elevated (normal would be up to 25 parts per billion). If this falls promptly after a discussion about adherence (or following admission for directly observed treatment), this suggests that the child was not taking their treatment correctly at home. A detailed discussion of the utility of FeNO in clinical practice is beyond the scope of this brief discussion. However, more details can be found in the draft NICE guidance on diagnosis and monitoring of asthma in adults, children and young people (published January 2015 (4)).

Syllabus Mapping

Respiratory

- Be able to assess, diagnose and manage wheezing illnesses

References

1. Brand PLP, Baraldi E, Bisgaard H et al. Definition, assessment and treatment of wheezing disorders in preschool children: An evidence-based approach. Eur Respir J 2008; 32: 1096–110.

2. British Thoracic Society Scottish Intercollegiate Guidelines Network. British guidelines on the management of asthma 2014 [cited 2014]. http://www.brit-thoracic.org.uk/document-library/clinical-information/asthma/btssign-asthma-guideline-2014/

3. Chan AHY et al. The effect of an electronic monitoring device with audiovisual reminder function on adherence to inhaled corticosteroids and school attendance in children with asthma: A randomised controlled trial. The Lancet Respiratory Medicine 2015: 3: 210–219.

4. http://www.nice.org.uk/guidance/gid-cgwave0640/documents/asthma-diagnosis-and-monitoring-draft-nice-guidance 2.

Chapter 31: A 3 year old boy who presents to the emergency department with bruises
Dr Jill Sussens, Dr Martin Hewitt

31

A 3 year old boy is brought to the emergency department by a police officer and a neighbour who had found him wandering in the street. The child is dishevelled and smells of urine. Both his parents attend a short while later and are antagonistic to each other. They are not married and do not live together. The child has been in the care of each of the parents and his maternal grandmother during the day. The maternal grandmother and a duty social worker both appear in the department.

The examination confirms the unkempt appearance of the child and identifies a bruise (caused by a hand slap) on the face of the child. This bruise is purple in colour. There are bruises on the spine. The child is otherwise well and is playing comfortably in the department. He plays comfortably with the mother, father and maternal grandmother. Both parents deny knowledge of the facial bruise.

Q1. Which of the following is the most appropriate placement for the child over the next 24 hours?

Select <u>one</u> answer only

A.   Admit the child to hospital
B.   Allow the child to go home to his maternal grandmother
C.   Allow the child to go home to his parents
D.   Allow the child to go to stay with the neighbour
E.   The social worker should place the child in emergency foster placement

Q2. Which of the following observations without an explanation suggests a non-accidental cause?

Select <u>one</u> answer only

A.   Bruise at the elbow
B.   Bruise on the pinna of ear
C.   Bruise on the forehead
D.   Bruise on the thigh
E.   Multiple bruises of different ages on the shins

Answers and Rationale

Q1. **E: The social worker should place the child in emergency foster placement**

Q2. **B: Bruise on pinna of ear**

The child in this story presents in a dishevelled and unkempt state with bruising that indicates physical abuse. It will require time to assess all the conflicting pieces of evidence. In the interim, the social care and medical team need to ensure the safety of this child. Both the parents and the maternal grandmother have all had responsibility for the child during the previous 24 hours and, consequently, any one of them may be responsible for the bruising. Although the neighbour is obviously caring, they are unable to receive the child as they have no legal responsibility and their background is not known. A place of safety needs to be found. This could be another family member approved by social care or an emergency foster placement. If such a placement is not possible, then the child may need to be admitted to the hospital while a safe place is found.

The position of bruising on the body needs to be related to the history given by the carer. Bruising below the knee is generally considered to be the result of normal activity in a young child. Bruises over bony prominences (such as knees, shoulders and the elbow) would be expected in accidental trauma. Bruising to the pinna is unusual and likely the result of a slap or a pinch. Bruising with a clear pattern, such as a slap mark, is clearly non-accidental (1, 2).

Robust safeguarding procedures that protect children and young people are paramount for any clinical team (3). These procedures are established by multidisciplinary teams with representatives from healthcare, social services and the police, and have to be consistent with the national legal framework. The UN Convention on the Rights of the Child defines a child as anyone who has not attained their 18th birthday, and this has been ratified by the UK Government.

Although each of the 4 UK nations has differing laws on child protection, they all apply these laws to those under 18 years of age. All 4 governments have established a legal framework that aims to provide protection to those under 18 years from physical, emotional and sexual abuse and from neglect.

Key individuals are appointed in health, social services and the police with a specific responsibility to ensure that the local police place child welfare at the centre of practice. This will include guidance to all in contact with the children on identifying those at risk, clear pathways of referral for concerns, and robust methods of investigating those referrals in a prompt and timely manner.

Where a child is presented to the medical staff in an acute setting with concerns about the potential causes of injury or insult, it is then incumbent on all to ensure that the child or young person is safe while a full history and examination are undertaken. The collection of such information can take time and requires the input from colleagues in social care and the police. It is vitally important to maintain comprehensive and contemporaneous notes, including identifiable quotes from differing parties and 'body map' illustrations that record any external lesions, including bruises. Medical photographs are invaluable and out-of-normal working hours can be performed by the police. Many units will provide pre-printed assessment packs to ensure all the relevant data is collected.

The assessment of bruising in children can be difficult and, in particular, the mechanism of causation can be open to differing interpretation. It is important to consider the potential range of alternative explanations for bruising in a child, including the possibility of a first presentation of an underlying pathological illness, such as leukaemia or clotting disorder (although even these children can still suffer physical abuse).

The extent and site of bruising needs to be placed in the context of the provided history – and there may be differing explanations given. The age and mobility of a child should be considered when reviewing the history. A study of 900 well children attending a 'well child' clinic found that only 0.6% of the children who were younger than 6 months and 1.7% of children younger than 9 months had any bruises. Increasing mobility brought the expected increase in bruising, with approximately 17% of infants who were cruising and 52% of children who were walking having obvious bruises (4).

Very young children with limited mobility are unlikely to incur bruising at any site and, consequently, any bruising in a non-mobile infant requires further thorough assessment in line with local safeguarding procedures (5, 6, 7). Children who have started to stand and walk are clearly at risk of falls and bumps as they establish their mobility skills.

Consequently, bruising should be expected at sites of impact, including shoulders, buttocks and head (particularly the forehead). However, an understanding of the extent of any fall is an important part of the history – a simple fall onto the buttocks from a standing position will not produce bruising in a child without an underlying clotting problem. Bruises to the face, ear and other protected body surfaces should raise concerns about physical abuse.

The shape of the bruises may indicate causation. Circular bruises suggest a human bite and will require advice from a forensic orthodontist to define the mouth size of the perpetrator. Linear marks might point to a hand slap (the linear appearance from the gap between the fingers, allowing small capillaries to rupture) or the use of a stick. The latter feature is suggestive of excessive chastisement and would be an offence under UK law, no matter the misdemeanour committed by the child. No parent, teacher or other adult is allowed to use unreasonable or excessive force.

The attempt to define the age of a bruise is a common request to clinicians from the police and social services, as this helps narrow down the pool of potential suspects. Multiple studies have been undertaken and all conclude that bruises cannot be accurately aged – no matter the background or seniority of the clinician (8)! The appearance of yellow pigmentation within bruises is not seen before 24 hours and generally only appears in bruises over 48 hours old.

Syllabus Mapping

Safeguarding

- Know the different presentations of non-accidental injury: physical, emotional, sexual, neglect and fabricated and induced illness and how to differentiate these from accidental injury, diseases and variations of normality

- Be able to assess and manage physical and emotional abuse and fabricated and induced illness

References

1. Pierce MC, Kaczor K, Aldridge S, O'Flynn J, Lorenz DJ. Bruising characteristics discriminating physical child abuse from accidental trauma. Pediatrics 2010; 125: 67–74.

2. Core Info. Cardiff Child Protection Systematic Reviews. http://www.core-info.cardiff.ac.uk/.

3. Child Protection Companion. Royal College of Paediatrics and Child Health, 2006.

4. Sugar NH, Taylor JA, Feldman KW. Bruises in infants and toddlers; Those who don't cruise rarely bruise. Archives of Pediatrics and Adolescent Medicine 1999; 153: 399–403.

5. Kemp AM, Dunstan F, Nuttall D, Hamilton M, Collins P, Maguire SA. Patterns of bruising in preschool children – A longitudinal study. Arch Dis Child 2015; 100: 426–431.

6. Carpenter RF. The prevalence and distribution of bruising in babies. Arch Dis Child 1999; 80: 363–366.

7. Pierce M, Smith S, Kaczor K. Bruising in infants: Those with a bruise may be abused. Pediatric Emergency Care 2009; 25: 845–847.

8. Bariciak ED, Plint AC, Gaboury I, Bennett S. Dating of bruises in children: An assessment of physician accuracy. Pediatrics 2003; 112: 804–807.

Chapter 32: A 12 year old boy who needs a small surgical procedure
Dr Jill Sussens, Dr Martin Hewitt

(32)

A 12 year old boy is seen in the clinic with his foster mother. He is in voluntary foster care and his mother has recently been sent to prison. He has a large skin tag on his ear and is being teased at school about it. He is keen to have this surgically removed and his foster mother is in agreement. His biological father died recently in a car crash, but he has met his paternal grandparents and they live nearby. His parents were not married.

Q1. Which of the following can give consent for any proposed surgery for this patient?

Select <u>one</u> answer only

A. Assigned social worker
B. Foster mother
C. Grandparents of the birth father
D. Mother
E. Senior paediatric surgeon

Q2. If the biological father had not died which of the following individuals would have parental responsibility regarding operative consent for this child?

Select <u>one</u> answer only

A. Assigned social worker (on behalf of local social services)
B. Biological father (named on the birth certificate in January 2004 but there has been no contact for 5 years)
C. Biological father (who was not married to mother at the time of birth and is not on the birth certificate)
D. Current partner of the mother (who has cared for the child for last 5 years)
E. Foster carer

Answers and Rationale

Q1. **D: Mother**
Q2. **B: Biological father (named on birth certificate in January 2004 but no contact for 5 years)**

Parental responsibility refers to the duties placed on an adult who has an explicit role in the care of a child.

A mother automatically has this responsibility for her child from birth, and this responsibility remains whatever the domestic or personal circumstances of the mother. It can only be removed if the mother voluntarily surrenders this role or if the responsibility is removed by a court order. The father of a child has parental responsibility if he is married to the mother of the child or is listed on the birth certificate after December 2003. This responsibility continues even if the parents subsequently divorce.

If the parents were not married at the time of birth, the father can only obtain the legal responsibility for his child by jointly registering the birth of the child with the mother (and thereby being named on the birth certificate) by marrying the mother, by obtaining a formal, legally recognised written agreement with the mother, or by asking a court of law to allocate such a responsibility. Same sex partners who were civil partners at the time of the treatment will both have parental responsibility.

Children may be placed into the care of foster parents on a voluntarily basis, and this is arranged through the local social services team. The parents, however, retain full legal responsibility for the child. Similarly, the child may be placed with a foster family following a court order and, in this situation, parental responsibility lies with the local authority who shares it with the parents (the mother would retain this until it was removed). Foster carers, therefore, have significant responsibility for the day-to-day care of the children in their care and make a wide range of decisions, but parental responsibility is not transferred to the foster carer. The carers must seek permission from those with parental responsibility for any significant interventions.

Families who adopt a child will be given the parental responsibility by the court ruling. The 2 parents named on the adoption application will have joint and equal responsibility, whether that is in a different-sex or same-sex relationship.

Consent is the process of giving permission for another individual to undertake a course of action that would otherwise be interpreted as battery and assault. Such consent is required for all medical interventions, although it does not necessarily need to be in a written form.

The transition from a dependent child who is unable to give consent to an independent adult who is capable of taking decisions on very complex options is different for different individuals, different backgrounds and different problems.

'Consent' and 'refusal to consent' are opposite views on the same question, but lead to different guidance for the patient and the clinician. They are seen as different entities within the legal statutes (1).

In order for a young person under 16 to be able to consent or to refuse consent, they must be deemed to have capacity – this implies they understand the nature, purpose and possible consequences of the investigations or treatments proposed, as well as the consequences of not having treatment.

Only if they are able to understand, retain, use and weigh this information and communicate their decision to others, can they consent to that investigation or treatment. Clearly, all relevant information has to be discussed before deciding whether or not a child or young person has the capacity to consent.

The General Medical Council states that the clinician must 'assess maturity and understanding on an individual basis and with regard to the complexity and importance of the decision to be made' (2).

Simple interventions may be understood and consent obtained in a child who may not be in a position to consent to a more complex and risky procedure. It is therefore the clinician who has to make this assessment of capacity to understand, and clear records must be kept.

Refusal of treatment by a young person requires more stringent checks and safeguards to be in place. If the refusal is not thought to be in the best interests of the young person, then the doctor may seek the consent of the parents. It may, however, be necessary to seek court approval, as such decisions may conflict with the human rights of the individual. It is possible, in some cases, for parents or the courts to overrule the decision of the young person, although the practicalities of implementing the decision may be difficult.

It is accepted that, in emergency situations, life-saving treatment can be given without consent as long as it is in the patient's best interests, and it is usual clinical practice that 2 senior clinicians make that decision.

Syllabus Mapping

Ethics and the Law

- Be able to apply legal rights of children and young people within the current UK legal framework

References

1. Palmer R, Gillespie G. Consent and capacity in children and young people. Arch Dis Child Edu Pract Ed 2014; 99: 2–7.

2. General Medical Council. 0–18 years: Guidance for all doctors, 2007.

Further Reading

Cave E, Stavrinides Z. Medical Practitioners, Adolescents and Informed Consent Project Final Report. University of Leeds, April 2013.

Ashteka CS, Hande A, Stallard E, Tuthill D. How much do junior staff know about common legal situations in paediatrics? Child Care Health Development 2007; 35: 631–634.

Working together to safeguard children: A guide to inter-agency working to safeguard and promote the welfare of children. HM Government 2015.

Chapter 33: An infant with diarrhoea and a rash
Dr Lucy Hinds

A 3 month old breastfed boy presents with a history of loose stools and a severe eczematous rash. He was born in the UK to Pakistani parents who are first cousins. On examination, his length and weight are on the 0.4th centiles. Apart from a severe rash, his examination is otherwise normal.

Investigations

Blood

Haemoglobin	96 g/l
White cell count	$4.0 \times 10^9/l$
neutrophils	$3.4 \times 10^9/l$
lymphocytes	$0.3 \times 10^9/l$
eosinophils	$0.5 \times 10^9/l$
Platelets	$178 \times 10^9/l$

Immunoglobulins

IgA	<0.07 g/dl (0.05–0.6)
IgG	1.0 g/dl (1.5–8.0)
IgM	0.1 g/dl (0.1–1.0)
IgE	200 U/l (<230)

Q1. Which of the following is the most likely diagnosis?

Select <u>one</u> answer only

A. Congenitally acquired HIV infection
B. Hyper IgE syndrome
C. Severe combined immune deficiency (SCID)
D. Wiskott-Aldrich syndrome
E. X-linked agammaglobulinaemia

Q2. Which of the following interventions is the most appropriate for this condition?

Select <u>one</u> answer only

A. Antiretroviral treatment
B. Bone marrow transplantation
C. Exclude cow's milk from the mother's diet
D. Systemic steroids
E. Topical steroids and emollients

Answers and Rationale

Q1.   C: Severe combined immune deficiency (SCID)
Q2.   B: Bone marrow transplantation

The history of diarrhoea, faltering growth and severe eczema-like rash is suggestive of a diagnosis of SCID, which is supported by the severe lymphopaenia. The parent's consanguinity makes an inherited autosomal recessive condition more likely. The diagnosis can be reinforced by the absence of a thymic shadow on a chest x-ray. SCID represents the most severe form of immunodeficiency and has an incidence of around 1 in 58,000 live births. A variety of inherited molecular defects prevent or severely impair T-cell and B-cell development and function, the most common of which is a mutation in the gamma chain of the interleukin (IL) receptors, a protein encoded on the X chromosome leading to X-linked SCID. SCID is a paediatric emergency because survival depends on early stem cell reconstitution, with bone marrow transplantation, which can be life-saving and, if successful, is curative. A lymphocyte count of less than 2.0×10^9/l on two occasions in infants should prompt the suspicion of SCID (1, 2).

Congenitally acquired HIV infection can present with faltering growth and diarrhoea and may be associated with pustular dermatitis. A baby presenting with evidence of such severe immune deficiency due to HIV would be expected to have a very low CD4 count, leading to a low total lymphocyte count. However, the prevalence of HIV infection in Pakistan is relatively low and this baby was born in the UK where mothers are tested for HIV infection during pregnancy, unless they specifically 'opt out' of screening (3).

X-linked agammaglobulinaemia (Bruton's disease) is an X-linked immunodeficiency caused by mutations that result in humoral immune deficiency manifested by the failure of B-cell maturation and very low levels of immunoglobulins IgA, IgG and IgM. They do not have cellular immune deficiency (1). Affected patients have absent tonsillar and adenoid tissue, as well as gut lymphoid tissue. These patients present early in childhood with recurrent respiratory tract infections, including pneumonia and sinusitis due to encapsulated bacteria, especially Streptococcus pneumoniae and Haemophilus influenzae. Diarrhoea is also a prominent symptom due to infection with organisms including Giardia and Campylobacter. Eczema is not usually a significant feature. Treatment is monthly intravenous or subcutaneous immunoglobulin therapy.

Dermatitis may be seen in other forms of primary immune deficiency, including Wiskott-Aldridge syndrome, which is a triad of eczema, immune deficiency and thrombocytopaenia. The platelet count in this case is normal, excluding Wiskott-Aldridge syndrome. The most effective intervention for a child with Wiskott-Aldridge syndrome would also be to proceed to a bone marrow transplantation. Other immune deficiencies that present with skin manifestations include hyper IgE syndrome (HIES) with eczema and skin abscesses. These patients have extremely high levels of IgE. Telangiectasia is a presenting feature of ataxia telangiectasia. Partial albinism with silvery grey hair is seen in Chediak-Higashi syndrome. Severe atopic eczema may present at 3 months of age, but would not typically be associated with loose stools and faltering growth. Eosinophilia would also be expected, rather than lymphopaenia. Cow's milk protein intolerance can present with diarrhoea and faltering growth even in breastfed infants (see chapter 12). It would, however, not usually be associated with lymphopaenia.

Syllabus Mapping

Infection Immunology and Allergy

* Know the causes and common presentations of vulnerability to infection including primary/secondary immunodeficiency and when to refer

References and Further Reading

1. Klein N, Neth O, Eisen S. Infection and Immunity. In: Gardiner M, Eisen S, Murphy C (eds). Training in Paediatrics. Oxford University Press: Oxford, 2009: 307–344.

2. Kwan A, Puck J. Newborn Screening for Severe Combined Immunodeficiency. Current Pediatrics Reports 2015; 3: 34–42.

3. Gennery AR, Cant AJ. Diagnosis of severe combined immunodeficiency. Journal of Clinical Pathology 2001; 54: 191–195.

Chapter 34: A 2 year old boy with persistent fever and a rash
Dr Robert Dinwiddie

(34)

A 2 year old boy presents to the emergency department with a 6-day history of sore throat, persistent fever and a rash. On examination, his temperature is 38.9°C, respiratory rate 28/minute and heart rate 120/minute. He is alert but miserable. He has conjunctival injection, his mouth and throat are acutely inflamed, his chest is clear and heart sounds normal, blood pressure 95/55 mmHg, his abdomen is soft and his neurological examination is normal. He has a morbilliform rash on his trunk and lower limbs and the swelling of his hands and feet.

Q1. Which of the following is the most likely diagnosis?

Select one answer only

A.   Hand, foot, and mouth disease
B.   Henoch-Schonlein purpura
C.   Kawasaki disease (KD)
D.   Measles
E.   Scarlet fever

Q2. Which of the following is the most serious potential complication?

Select one answer only

A.   Acute glomerulonephritis
B.   Aseptic meningitis
C.   Bleeding due to thrombocytopaenia
D.   Coronary artery aneurysms
E.   Toxic shock

Q3. Which of the following treatment regimens is the most effective in preventing the most important long-term complication at this stage?

Select one answer only

A.   Aspirin
B.   IV immunoglobulin
C.   IV methylprednisolone
D.   Anti-TNF-alpha (infliximab)
E.   Ciclosporin

Answers and rationale

Q1. **C: Kawasaki disease (KD)**
Q2. **D: Coronary artery aneurysms**
Q3. **B: IV Immunoglobulin**

This boy has Kawasaki disease (KD) based on his age, history and the physical signs, including persistent fever, conjunctival injection, oral mucositis, morbilliform rash and oedema of his hands and feet. Hand foot and mouth disease, caused by Coxsackie viruses, is unlikely because it would not usually cause this degree of systemic illness, the hands and feet would have vesicles rather than swelling, and the oral inflammation also commonly results in vesicles on the tongue. Henoch-Schönlein purpura can also cause oedema of the hands and feet in the early stages but the rash would be purpuric rather than morbilliform. Measles would obviously cause a morbilliform rash and conjunctivitis but the high fever does not usually last for 6 days. Scarlet fever also presents with sore throat and fever but the rash, which is erythematous, and the blanching starts in the axillae and groins. Desquamation in scarlet fever occurs during the second week of the illness, most commonly affecting the face, trunk and limbs.

KD is the second most common vasculitic disease of childhood after Henoch-Schönlein purpura (1- 3). KD is the most common cause of acquired heart disease in developed countries (4). The disease has a worldwide distribution with a preponderance of males and an ethnic bias toward Asian, especially Japanese, children. The incidence in the UK is 8.1 in 100,000, whereas in Japan, it is 138 in 100,000. It probably represents an aberrant inflammatory response to an as yet unidentified pathogen or pathogens. It is associated with systemic vasculitis particularly affecting the coronary arteries.

The disease occurs in 3 parts: the acute phase (days 1–10), the subacute phase (days 11–25) and the convalescent phase. Diagnostic criteria include a fever of up to 39°C for at least 5 days, together with any 4 of the following: rash (diffused non-vesicular and polymorphic), conjunctivitis which is bilateral and non-ulcerating, oral mucositis with a strawberry tongue, erythema and the cracking of lips and tongue, cervical adenopathy (usually unilateral and >1.5 cm in size), erythema, and oedema of the peripheral extremities in the first week (2). In the subacute phase, peeling of the skin occurs on the fingers and toes and thrombocytosis is common.

An incomplete form, more common in infants, is also seen with fever but with fewer of the other criteria present. This can lead to delay in diagnosis. This form of KD is also associated with a higher incidence of coronary artery aneurysms. An important differential diagnosis is acute rheumatic fever, which can present with many similar features (2). However, in these cases, there is usually evidence of recent acute infection with group A beta haemolytic Streptococcus with positive anti-Streptococcal ASO antibody titres and elevated anti-DNase B levels.

Glomerulonephritis is not a feature of KD, although sterile pyuria is described. Meningism is not a major complicating feature of KD, although irritability is not uncommon and white blood cells may be seen in the cerebrospinal fluid (CSF). Thrombocytopaenia leading to purpura and bleeding is not seen in KD despite the mucositis and the oral and dermatological features. The rash is typically non-purpuric, unlike that seen in Henoch-Schönlein purpura. The most important complications are cardiac, including myocarditis, but especially the development of coronary artery aneurysms that can have lethal short-term and long-term complications. Toxic shock, which can present clinically with similar features including fever, oral mucositis, a macular rash and desquamation of the hands and feet, is a complication of bacterial toxins particularly from *Staphylococcus aureus* and *Streptococcus pyogenes*.

KD leads to the formation of coronary artery aneurysms in as many as 15–25% of untreated cases. The incidence is higher in young infants who present with 'incomplete' KD. The aneurysms may be small but, in some cases, progress to significant dilatation or even giant aneurysms >8 mm in size. These can lead to acute coronary artery thrombosis or stenosis with the risk of cardiac ischaemia many months or even years later.

Routine treatment includes aspirin, but the most effective regime is intravenous immunoglobulin (IVIG) (combined with aspirin) that is started during the acute phase of the illness. This regime reduces the severity of the coronary artery lesions but not their long-term outcome. Corticosteroids, either by the oral or intravenous route, are widely, but not universally, used. They are particularly useful in resistant cases. Recent trials of anti-TNF-alpha (infliximab) have shown significant reduction in fever and shorter hospital stay, but no reduction in the incidence of coronary artery complications (4). Ciclosporin has been used in resistant cases but, so far, without evidence of reduction in long-term complications.

The recurrence rate is approximately 2%. Long-term follow-up for those with coronary artery complications is required and may need to be lifelong in the more severe cases.

Syllabus Mapping

Musculoskeletal

- Be able to assess, diagnose and manage vasculitic disorders with appropriate referral

Cardiology

- Know the cardiac complications of other system disorders

References and Further Reading

1. Eleftheriou D, Levin M, Shingadia D, Tulloh R, Klein NJ, Borgan PA. Management of Kawasaki disease. Arch Dis Ch 2014; 99: 74–83

2. Gardiner M, Eisen S, Murphy C. Rheumatic fever and Kawasaki disease. In: Gardiner M, Eisen S, Murphy C (eds). Training in Paediatrics. Oxford University Press: Oxford, 2009:86-87.

3. Harnden A, Tulloh R, Burgner D. Kawasaki disease. BMJ 2014; 349: 35–37.

4. Lin MT, Sun LI, Wu ET, Wang JK, Lue HC, Wu MH. Acute and late coronary outcomes in 1,073 patients with Kawasaki disease with and without intravenous immunoglobulin therapy. Arch Dis Ch 2015; 100: 542-547.

Chapter 35: A newborn baby with a petechial rash
Dr Mithilesh Lal, Professor Win Tin

(35)

A male infant with a birthweight of 3.4 kg is noted to have a widespread petechial rash at about 24 hours of age. He was born at term by a normal delivery to a primiparous Caucasian mother. The maternal record does not indicate any antenatal problems. The baby was given oral vitamin K (1 mg) at birth. There are no other concerns raised by the mother or the midwife, who is looking after him on the post-natal ward, and he is said to be breastfeeding well.

Clinically, the baby appears well, and there is no pallor, jaundice or any signs of active bleeding. His temperature is 37.1°C, his heart rate 140/minute, and his respiratory rate 40/minute. His liver is just palpable, but there is no splenomegaly.

Investigations

Blood

Haemoglobin	149 g/l
White cell count	24.9 x 10^9/l
Platelets	11 x 10^9/l
PT	17 seconds
APPT	45 seconds

Q1: What is the most likely diagnosis?

Select <u>one</u> answer only

A. Congenital CMV infection
B. Congenital leukaemia
C. Maternal immune thrombocytopaenic purpura
D. Neonatal alloimmune thrombocytopaenia (NAIT)
E. Vitamin K deficiency bleeding

Q2: What is the most appropriate specific management of this condition?

Select <u>one</u> answer only

A. Human platelet antigens (HPA) compatible donor platelet concentrate
B. IVIG infusion
C. Oral prednisolone
D. Packed cell blood transfusion
E. Random donor platelet concentrate

Answer and Rationale

Q1. **D: Neonatal alloimmune thrombocytopaenia (NAIT)**
Q2. **A: Human platelet antigens (HPA) compatible donor platelet concentrate**

Incidence of severe thrombocytopaenia in term newborns is reported to be 1 in 1,000, and by far the most common cause in well infants is antibodies to HPA (1). In comparison, preterm infants are more likely to have low platelets due to infection or placental insufficiency. Of the 28 HPA systems and 34 alloantigens, HPA-1a (80%) and 5b (15%) are most common in Caucasians. Such alloantigens are most abundant in platelets but can also be expressed in other haematopoietic cells.

Maternal alloantibodies of the IgG type cross the placenta, bind to fetal platelets and cause thrombocytopaenia. The immune mechanism of NAIT is similar to Rh haemolytic disease except that it can present during first pregnancy (over 50% of cases). It remains under-diagnosed in the absence of any antenatal screening. Since NAIT is due to maternal sensitisation from fetal platelet-specific antigens, the maternal platelet count remains normal and there are no maternal risks, but the fetal platelet count is low and there are significant risks to the fetus during pregnancy and delivery.

Maternal autoantibodies can be seen in immune thrombocytopaenic purpura, systemic lupus erythematosus and drug-induced thrombocytopaenia (2).

In these conditions, in contrast to NAIT, the maternal platelet count is low and there is less risk to the fetus during pregnancy and delivery. The maternal risk in such cases will depend upon the degree of thrombocytopaenia.

It is difficult to predict the severity of NAIT based on any tests or antibody titres and, therefore, antibody titre is not performed routinely. NAIT should be suspected if any of the following criteria are present:

- Fetal or neonatal thrombocytopaenia
- Fetal intracranial haemorrhage, hydrocephalus, ventriculomegaly or cerebral cysts
- Unexplained fetal anaemia
- Recurrent, unexplained first trimester miscarriages
- Family history of NAIT
- Clinical evidence of bleeding in the fetus or newborn

Typical presentation includes a well-term, newborn baby with a widespread petechial rash at, or a few hours after, birth. Ecchymoses may be present; visceral haemorrhage, including intracranial haemorrhage, is uncommon. There may not be any significant maternal medical history or antenatal history. Clinical assessment is not suggestive of infection, congenital anomalies or disseminated intravascular coagulation.

Full blood count will indicate isolated thrombocytopaenia with normal red and white blood cell lines. Laboratory confirmation requires the presence of maternal HPA alloantibodies that react to the platelet-specific antigen of the father and infant but not the mother. Initial blood tests in both parents, if available, are sufficient for confirmation of NAIT.

All infants of a homozygous father will be affected, but only 50% of those who are heterozygous for the relevant HPA antigen. Antenatal HPA typing of the fetus can now be carried out from amniocentesis if a previous sibling was affected.

Management during pregnancy depends on the outcome of previous pregnancies, severity of thrombocytopaenia, specificity of HPA antibodies and the zygosity of the father. General precautions such as avoidance of non-steroidal anti-inflammatory drugs and fetal scalp electrodes, consideration for a Caesarean section and liaison with a blood bank for HPA compatible platelets apply.

An IVIG infusion at weekly intervals beyond 20 to 28 weeks of gestation is the first-line management. Double dose IVIG with corticosteroids may be tried if the response is poor. Fetal blood sampling with transfusion of compatible platelets still carries significant risk of morbidity and mortality.

During the neonatal period, a HPA-compatible donor platelet concentrate is used for treatment, and usually a single transfusion is adequate. Random donor platelets may be used on clinical grounds if serious bleeding happens while waiting for HPA-1a-5b negative platelets. IVIG is not the first-line treatment, but can produce a predictable increase in platelet count in 75% of cases after 24 to 48 hours of administration.

Syllabus Mapping

Haematology and Oncology

- Be able to assess, diagnose and manage coagulation disorders, hypercoagulable states, purpura and bruising

Reference and Further Reading

1. Lucas G. Neonatal Alloimmune Thrombocytopenia – Clinical guideline 272/1.4 Effective 30/10/14. http://hospital.blood.co.uk/resources/clinical-guidelines/NAIT.

2. Blickstein I, Friedman S. Fetal effects of autoimmune disease. In: Martin RJ, Fanaroff AA, Walsh MC (eds). Fanaroff and Martin's Neonatal-Perinatal Medicine: Diseases of the Fetus and Infant, 10th edition. Elsevier Saunders, 2015: 305–8.

Chapter 36: A 3 year old boy with a periocular rash
Dr Neil Rogers

A 3 year old Asian boy presents with a unilateral facial rash for the previous 10 days. He has no significant medical history and is otherwise well. There is no relevant family history. He is meeting all his milestones. He is on no regular medication. His visual acuity is normal, the eye has minimal conjunctival hyperaemia and there is no photophobia.

Image 36.1

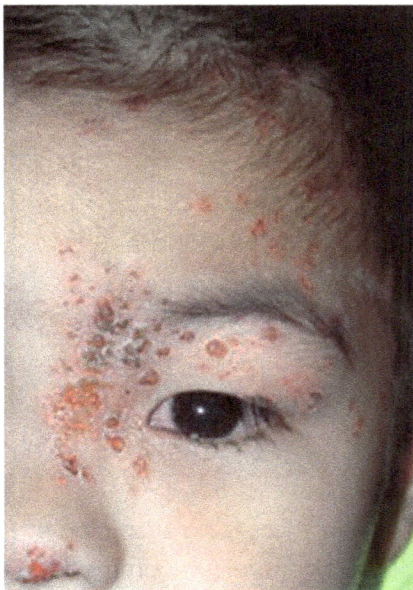

Q1. Which of the following is the most likely predisposing factor?

Select <u>one</u> answer only

A.   Chicken pox in the first year of life
B.   Contact with a child who has eczema herpeticum
C.   Haematological malignancy
D.   Recent immunisation against varicella-zoster (VZ) virus
E.   Systemic immune deficiency

Q2. Which of the following is the most likely long-term ocular outcome for this child?

Select <u>one</u> answer only

A.   Corneal blindness
B.   Glaucoma
C.   Normal visual acuity
D.   Uveitic cataract
E.   Zoster retinitis

Answers and Rationale

Q1.   A: Chicken pox in the first year of life
Q2.   C: Normal visual acuity

The picture demonstrates herpes zoster affecting the ophthalmic dermatome of the trigeminal nerve, including the nasociliary branch with lesions on the tip of the nose (Hutchinson's sign). The most important predisposing factor is having contracted chicken pox within the first year of life. Eczema herpeticum is caused by the herpes simplex virus, which does not cause an eruption in a dermatomal distribution. Children with haematological malignancy and immune deficiencies are at risk of developing herpes zoster ophthalmicus (HZO), but do not form a large contingent of those with HZO (1, 2). Recent immunisation against the VZ virus is not a risk factor.

Most children do not develop any long-term ocular complications from HZO, and have normal visual acuity. Some degree of corneal opacification occurs in approximately 20% of children, but corneal blindness would be an uncommon complication in fit and healthy children with HZO. Glaucoma and post-herpetic neuralgia are much more common in the elderly with HZO, but rarely occur in children. Zoster retinitis is a rare complication in the immunocompromised.

Herpes viruses are DNA viruses. HZO describes a zoster infection (shingles) affecting the ophthalmic division of the trigeminal nerve, with the potential to affect any ocular or periocular structure, e.g. scleritis, keratitis, uveitis. The open eye with white sclera is a strong indication that the eye is not involved in this particular child. This is most likely to occur in otherwise healthy children who have previously had chicken pox in infancy. Those with pre-existing immune compromise or systemic malignancy are at increased risk of developing HZO, but form a small proportion of children with the condition (3).

The prognosis is excellent in most cases and further investigation is unnecessary where there is no suspicion of any underlying condition. However, treatment with an antiviral drug such as aciclovir is generally recommended in HZO due to the risk of eye involvement. Ideally, treatment would be started in the first 72 hours of infection.

Skin depigmentation may occur later in the area of the vesicles.

Syllabus Mapping

Ophthalmology

* Be able to assess, diagnose and manage ophthalmological conditions including glaucoma and papilloedema and know when to refer

References and Further Reading

1. De Freitas D, Martins EN, Adan C, Alvarenga LS, Pavan-Langston D. Herpes Zoster Ophthalmicus in Otherwise Healthy Children. Am J Ophthalmol 2006; 142: 393–399.

2. Feder HM Jr, Hoss DM. Herpes zoster in otherwise healthy children. Pediatr Infect Dis J 2004 May; 23: 451–457; quiz 458–60.

3. Grote V, von Kries R, Rosenfeld E, Belohradsky BH, Liese J. Immunocompetent Children Account for the Majority of Complications in Childhood Herpes Zoster. J Infect Dis 2007; 196: 1455–1458.

Chapter 37: A toddler with acute cough and wheeze
Dr Rob Primhak

37

A 2 year old girl presents to the emergency department with an acute wheeze and breathlessness. She has had a runny nose for 4 days, but was otherwise well until 3 hours prior to her attendance, when she started coughing and wheezing and became breathless.

She has 2 older siblings who have also had recent colds. Her father suffered from asthma, and one sibling has a history of wheezing with colds.

On examination, she is afebrile, with a heart rate of 120/minute and a respiratory rate of 30/minute. She has a widespread expiratory wheeze, and frequent paroxysms of cough. Her oxygen saturation is 94% in air.

She is given 3 salbutamol nebulisers in the first hour, without any improvement.

Her chest imaging is shown below.

Figure 37.1: Chest image

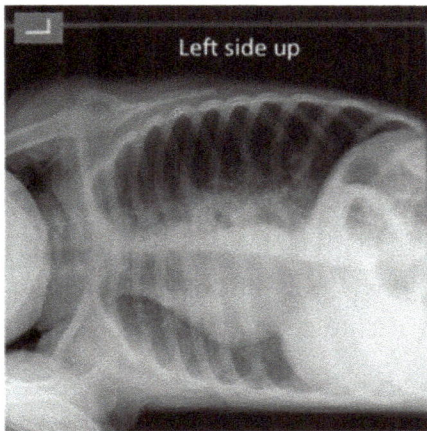

Figure 37.2: Chest image

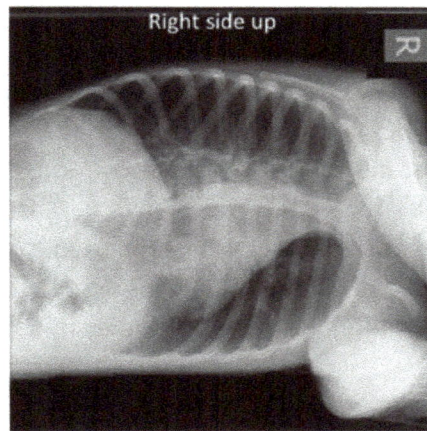

Q1. What is the next appropriate management step?

Select <u>one</u> answer only

A.   IM adrenaline 0.01 ml/kg of 1:1000 strength
B.   IV magnesium sulfate bolus
C.   IV salbutamol 15 microgm/kg over 5 minutes
D.   Nebulised ipratropium bromide
E.   Prednisolone 1 mg/kg orally
F.   Rigid bronchoscopy
G.   Start a macrolide antibiotic

Answers and Rationale

Q1.   F: Rigid bronchoscopy

Most episodes of wheezing in 2 year olds are caused by viral episodic wheeze, and the fact that the patient has recently suffered a cold would support this diagnosis. However, there are several atypical features. The first is the abrupt onset of wheezing. This would suggest either an anaphylactic episode, or a foreign body inhalation.

The failure to respond to nebulised salbutamol is another feature against the diagnosis of a viral episodic wheeze. However, in this case, the other striking clue is in the decubitus x-rays. Since the intrathoracic airways expand during inspiration and collapse during expiration, air trapping tends to occur beyond a bronchial foreign body. In older children, an expiratory film will demonstrate a failure of the obstructed lung to deflate. In a young child, an expiratory film may not be possible as they are unable to hold their breath in expiration. The films in the present case show normal deflation of the dependent right lung when the left side is up, but no deflation of the dependent left lung when the right side is up. This is strongly suggestive of a left main bronchus obstruction. This technique has also been used with CT scans to evaluate air trapping in less cooperative patients (1).

It should be noted that the air trapping and expiratory wheezing seen in the first or second day of a foreign body is usually followed by resorption atelectasis and suppuration if it is not removed promptly. Bronchiectasis may follow a foreign body aspiration, particularly when the foreign body is organic, or when there is delay in removal (2).

Although there was no observed episode of aspiration in the history, this is not uncommon in childhood foreign body inhalation. In a series of 70 children with confirmed foreign body aspiration, sudden onset of choking or coughing followed by persistent cough was the most common feature in the history. Localised wheezing was observed in only 30%, and localised reduction in air entry in 62%, while 25% were felt to have diffuse wheezing (3). Although a sudden onset of coughing in association with localised wheeze and reduced air entry was highly suggestive of a foreign body, this triad was present in only 15% of patients. It should also be noted that less than 10% of inhaled foreign bodies in children are radio-opaque.

Points that should make the clinician suspect an inhaled foreign body are a history of choking or abrupt onset of cough in a previously well child, localised wheeze with or without reduced air entry, early radiology showing localised hyperinflation, and a later radiology showing significant localised volume loss.

Rigid bronchoscopy is preferred to flexible bronchoscopy in the diagnosis and removal of foreign bodies from the airway. Although it is feasible to remove a foreign body with a flexible bronchoscopy, it is far easier to use the larger access channel of a rigid instrument.

The other answers offered in the question relate to the management of acute wheezing, which is poorly responsive to nebulised salbutamol. Intramuscular adrenaline would be an appropriate treatment of an anaphylactic reaction, if that was a likely cause. Nebulised ipratropium is helpful as additive treatment in severe wheezing, and magnesium sulfate, salbutamol and aminophylline are all appropriate second-line treatments in severe asthma (4). Magnesium sulfate is becoming the first option to be used in this situation in view of its low side-effect profile (5). Oral steroids, such as prednisolone, have been shown to be ineffective in preschool children with viral induced wheeze (6), but may still be used in severe attacks where initial treatment is unhelpful. Macrolide antibiotics are helpful in atypical pneumonia with wheeze caused by Chlamydia or Mycoplasma, but these are less likely aetiologies in this case.

Syllabus Mapping

Respiratory

- Be able to assess, diagnose and manage wheezing illnesses

References and Further Reading

1. Choi SJ, Choi BK, Kim HJ et al. Lateral decubitus HRCT: A simple technique to replace expiratory CT in children with air trapping. Pediatric Radiology 2002; 32(3): 179–82. PubMed PMID: 12164350.

2. Karakoc F, Karadag B, Akbenlioglu C et al. Foreign body aspiration: What is the outcome? Pediatr Pulmonol 2002; 34(1): 30–6. PubMed PMID: 12112794.

3. Midulla F, Guidi R, Barbato A et al. Foreign body aspiration in children. Pediatrics International 2005; 47(6): 663–8.

4. British Thoracic Society and Scottish Intercollegiate Guidelines Network. British guidelines on the management of asthma. 2014. https://www.brit-thoracic.org.uk/document-library/clinical-information/asthma/btssign-asthma-guideline-2014/.

5. Lyttle MD, O'Sullivan R, Doull I et al. Variation in treatment of acute childhood wheeze in emergency departments of the United Kingdom and Ireland: An international survey of clinician practice. Archives of Disease in Childhood 2015; 100(2): 121–125.

6. Panickar, J et al. Oral prednisolone for preschool children with acute virus-induced wheezing. New England Journal of Medicine 2009; 360(4): 329–338.

Chapter 38: Poor diabetes control
Dr Joanna Walker

A 13 year old girl with type 1 diabetes is seen for an annual medical review in a diabetes outpatient clinic with both her parents. She was diagnosed at age 5 and continues to share care with them. Her parents give the injections in her thighs and she rotates between all other available injection sites. She has yet to start her periods. She catches the bus to school and then walks home with her friends. She has occasional hypoglycaemic episodes (hypos) which she recognises and manages appropriately. They attend the clinic regularly, at least 4 times every year, and she has annual retinal screenings. She is using a multiple daily insulin injection (MDII) regime, having tried but rejected a trial of a continuous subcutaneous insulin infusion (insulin pump) a couple of years previously. She injects 28 units of insulin detemir (long-acting) before bed, and 1 unit of soluble insulin for every 10 g of carbohydrate at mealtimes and with snacks.

On examination, she looks well and her height is following the 75th–91st centiles and her weight is on the 75th centile. She has some lumps at her injection sites, especially on either side of her umbilicus. Her blood pressure is 107/73 mmHg. She has reached breast and pubic hair stage 3.

Her annual review blood samples (taken prior to the clinic) show no evidence of thyroid or coeliac disease and her urine albumin to creatinine ratio (ACR) is normal. Her glycated haemoglobin (HbA$_1$c) is 67 mmol/mol (8.3%) compared with 52 mmol/mol (6.9%) at her appointment 3 months ago.

Table 38.1: Daily finger-prick blood glucose estimations (mmol/l)

Day	Before breakfast	Post breakfast	Before lunch	Post lunch	Before dinner	Post dinner	Before bed
Mon	8.6		10.5		6.7		
Tues				2.3			
Weds	7.9		9.4		14.5		10.5
Thurs	10.4					3.7	
Fri					5.6		
Sat	9.7		7.6	8.3			
Sun		10.4	5.4				
Mon	6.8						7.8
Tues			3.2		13.5		12.4
Weds	8.8						
Thurs			4.6				
Fri					5.2		6.9
Sat	11.3		13.7				
Sun		5.5					5.7

Q1. What advice would you give the family as the first step to improve her HbA$_1$c?

Select <u>one</u> answer only

A. Consider another trial of an insulin pump
B. Increase the evening dose of insulin detemir
C. Increase the ratio of insulin to carbohydrate (CHO) at mealtimes from 1 unit/10 g CHO to 1 unit/7.5 g CHO
D. Monitor blood glucose levels with a continuous subcutaneous glucose monitor
E. Remove the evening snack she has before going to bed

Q2. What is the likeliest cause for the deterioration in her HbA$_1$c?

Select <u>one</u> answer only

A. Eating snacks without giving insulin
B. Injecting into lumpy injection sites
C. Insulin resistance associated with puberty
D. Poor adherence to insulin treatment
E. Psychological difficulties in managing her diabetes

Answers and Rationale

Q1.   **B: Increase the evening dose of insulin detemir**
Q2.   **C: Insulin resistance associated with puberty**

The emphasis in recent years in the management of type 1 diabetes in children and young adults has focused on tightening control of blood glucose levels – changes that are reflected in the 2015 NICE guidelines (1). The aim is to achieve near normoglycaemia and, thereby, an HbA_1c level near the normal range (target 46 mmol/mol – 6.8%) in the hope of further reducing the long-term risks associated with this difficult diagnosis. This control is usually best achieved by intensive insulin management (MDII or pump therapy) from diagnosis, accompanied by carbohydrate counting. Perfection is impossible, but the aim is to achieve as many as possible glucose levels within 4.0–6.9 mmol/l.

When assessing a series of results, we look for patterns. The obvious pattern here is that this girl's glucose levels are high first thing in the morning. She is already injecting for snacks, so cutting out the one she has before bed will not influence this. Increasing her detemir to reduce her morning glucose levels may well be enough to improve some of her daytime levels without having to change the insulin to carbohydrate ratios, and this should happen first. She might need to alter the ratios in due course, but giving more soluble insulin as well as increasing the detemir might precipitate more daytime hypos.

If a pattern is not clear, it might be worth considering one of the newer technologies, such as continuous subcutaneous glucose monitoring, but this is not currently recommended for all children and young people with type 1 diabetes. It may be particularly valuable in children with frequent, disabling hypos and/or an inability to recognise or communicate them. There is no current evidence that insulin pumps significantly improve overall control compared with MDII, and there is plenty of scope to adjust her current regime first. There is no best way to manage type 1 diabetes and much depends on patient and family preference after discussion with the multidisciplinary team.

All the answers to Question 2 are possible.

Puberty is a time when many young people struggle to accept the diagnosis of type 1 diabetes, the restrictions to freedom it imposes, and the growing awareness of their future health prospects, which are often poor. Sharing information at regular meetings of the multidisciplinary team (including psychologists) involved in the tailored education and support of these patients and their families becomes even more important (1).

It is crucial to focus on the minutiae of insulin regimes to improve worsening control risks and not miss the 'messages' transmitted by these patients about the psychological and social difficulties so many of them encounter, which they have in common with young people with other chronic disorders. Having to inject with every snack they eat means that many of them regularly miss insulin, especially when out with their friends; they have more pressing priorities than carbohydrate counting and girls in particular may opt to control their weight by reducing insulin doses.

They avoid hypos by omitting or reducing insulin doses because hypos are unpleasant and their behaviour during them risks ridicule. As a result, the incidence of diabetic ketoacidosis (DKA) increases during this phase and is still a cause of death, especially in adolescent patients with suboptimal control. Death is usually due to cerebral oedema probably associated with excess intravenous fluids and/or a too rapid drop in blood glucose.

All children and young adults with DKA should be managed according to the UK national guidelines (2), the principles of which are not overestimating dehydration and shock, slow steady rehydration over 48–72 hours, delayed introduction of insulin by 1–2 hours after the start of any intravenous fluids, and close attention to detail with a senior review.

However, this girl seems to be doing her very best to manage her diabetes, well supported by her family. It is important to not jump to conclusions that this must be typical teenage behaviour. Most of her levels are reasonable and she has previously had excellent control. During puberty, there is reduced insulin sensitivity in all young people, compared with pre- and post-puberty, whether or not they have diabetes.

This insulin resistance is not completely understood but is due, in part, to the counterregulatory hormones, growth hormone and insulin-like growth factor 1 (IGF-1), which work against the action of insulin and are secreted at elevated levels during puberty to promote rapid growth and development (growth hormone secretion doubles during puberty). Insulin sensitivity drops by 25–30% in children with diabetes, so insulin requirements rise sharply. This girl's decline in control and need for higher doses of insulin are almost certainly the result of this physiological change.

Syllabus Mapping

Diabetes Mellitus

- Be able to assess, diagnose and manage diabetes and its complications including diabetic ketoacidosis

References and Further Reading

1. NICE guidelines (NG18). Diabetes (type 1 and type 2) in children and young people: diagnosis and management. Published date: August 2015.

2. http://www.bsped.org.uk/clinical/docs/DKAguideline.pdf

Chapter 39: A rotavirus vaccine trial
Dr Robert Dinwiddie

(39)

Study: An assessment of the efficacy and tolerability of a newly developed low-cost human-bovine (116E) rotavirus vaccine in low-resource urban and rural settings in India.

Methods: A randomised double-blind, placebo-controlled trial was carried out in 3 urban and rural sites in India between March 2011 and November 2102, where rotavirus immunisation is not currently available. Infants aged 6–7 weeks were randomly assigned to receive either 3 oral doses of the human-bovine vaccine (116E) or placebo at ages 6–7 weeks, 10 weeks and 14 weeks. The primary outcome was the incidence of severe rotavirus gastroenteritis.

Findings: 4,354 infants received the 116E vaccine and 2,187 received the placebo.

71 events of severe rotavirus gastroenteritis were reported in 4,752 person-years in the vaccine group compared with 76 events in the 2,360 person-years in the placebo group. Overall vaccine efficiency in the vaccinated group was 56.4% (95% confidence interval (CI) 36.6–70.1) in the first year of life. Six cases of intussusception were recorded in the vaccine group and 2 in the placebo group. Twenty-five (<1%) infants in the vaccine group and 17 (<1%) in the placebo group died. No death was regarded as being related to the vaccine.

Adapted from Lancet 2014; 383: 2136–2143.

Q1. From the data shown above, which of the following statements comparing the vaccinated group to the placebo group is correct?

Select <u>one</u> answer only

A.   A vaccine efficacy rate of 53.6% is unlikely to have substantial health benefits in developing countries
B.   Intussusception was significantly more common in vaccinated infants
C.   Rotavirus vaccination in infancy reduces the incidence of infection in children aged 2 years or more
D.   There was a higher mortality rate in the vaccine treated group
E.   Vaccinated infants had a significantly reduced incidence of severe rotavirus gastroenteritis in the first year of life

Q2. Which of the following general statements regarding rotavirus vaccines is correct?

Select <u>one</u> answer only

A.   A parenterally delivered vaccine would give greater protection
B.   An equivalent health benefit is likely in developed countries
C.   Comparison of the new vaccine to placebo, rather than other currently available vaccines, is the appropriate methodology for this study
D.   Rotavirus vaccines should not be co-administered with other vaccines
E.   This vaccine virus is unlikely to be transmitted to close contacts

Answers and Rationale

Q1. **E: Vaccinated infants had a significantly reduced incidence of severe rotavirus gastroenteritis in the first year of life**

Q2. **C: Comparison of the new vaccine to placebo, rather than other currently available vaccines, is the appropriate methodology for this study**

The vaccine efficacy rate and 95% confidence intervals quoted in the abstract demonstrate that there is a statistically significant difference in the incidence of rotavirus infection between the vaccinated and placebo groups in infants. In developing countries, even a vaccine efficacy rate of 56.3% is likely to have significant health benefits in this age group. Intussusception was not shown to be an increased risk for infants vaccinated in this study (1.37 in 1,000 versus 0.91 in 1,000) although this has been suggested as a possible complication in previous studies (1, 2). There is no data in this report to show that the vaccine reduced infection in children aged 2 years or over. The data quoted also shows that there is no increased mortality in the vaccinated group.

Rotavirus infection is the most common cause of severe dehydrating gastroenteritis in developing countries. India has the most rotavirus deaths in the world, estimated at 75,000 to 122,000 per year (3). In addition, it results in 400,000 to 800,000 hospital admissions per year (3). A cheap, safe, easily available, oral vaccine is required for use in countries such as this. At present, there are 2 other effective live attenuated rotavirus vaccines generally available, but even at their UNICEF-subsidised price of $3.50 per child, this inhibits their widespread use in low-income countries.

The most appropriate way to study a new vaccine in these epidemiological circumstances (low-income countries) is to compare the new vaccine to placebo. As already mentioned, the currently available vaccines are significantly more expensive, are not presently being used in this study setting, and have not been shown to be any more effective than this one. Other relevant points are that rotavirus is a gut-mediated infection, so mucosal immunity is vital to its efficacy, making an oral vaccine preferable to a parenteral one. Infants in developed countries are more likely to be intrinsically healthier, with better growth and weight gain for their age; thus, it is likely that a rotavirus infection in this population will have less severe health consequences and complications. Previous studies have demonstrated that rotavirus vaccines can safely be co-administered with several other vaccines (4). Rotavirus vaccine contains live virus, so it can readily be transmitted to other contacts, especially where basic hygiene standards are poor.

This study represents a unique partnership for the development of a low-cost vaccine between governmental agencies, international donors and an emerging local vaccine manufacturer (2). The virus chosen (116E) is a combination of naturally occurring strains containing 1 bovine rotavirus gene and 10 human rotavirus genes. It had previously been shown to readily and asymptomatically infect hospital neonates born in Delhi (1). The study performed was a double-blind, placebo-controlled randomised trial which is an entirely appropriate investigation into the efficacy of a new vaccine such as this one. Infants were randomised in a 2:1 ratio using a block size of 12. Block randomisation in this way eliminates possible allocation bias, which can imbalance treated versus placebo groups if larger, completely random allocation is used. This study also focused on 3 sites – Delhi (urban), Pune (rural) and Vellore (urban and rural). This enabled it to reflect the realistic possibility of the implementation of any positive results in a variety of population settings. This is another reason why randomisation using block allocation was appropriate in these particular circumstances.

The efficacy of this and other rotavirus vaccines is of the order of 50–60%. Due to the huge disease burden of this illness, even at this level, the healthcare benefits are likely to be substantial (2). One practical problem, however, will be in the infrastructure required to deliver 3 directly observed doses of this vaccine to such large numbers of children in low-income countries. Studies such as this have involved large numbers of research-funded vaccine administrators on the ground. In order for this to be replicated in real life, a major infrastructure of community-based vaccine administrators will need to be funded and put in place at a national level. This will require the governments of countries such as India to make this a major health priority for the future.

Syllabus Mapping

Science of Practice

- Be able to interpret a research paper or systemic review appropriately

References and Further Reading

1. Bhandari N, Rongsen-Chandola T, Bavdekar A et al. Efficacy of monovalent human-bovine rotavirus vaccine in Indian infants: A randomised double-blind placebo-controlled trial. Lancet 2014; 383: 2136–2143.

2. Mahdi SA, Parashar UD. 116E rotavirus development: A successful alliance. Lancet 2014; 383: 2106–2107.

3. Bhan MK, Glass RI, Ella KM et al. Team science and the creation of a novel rotavirus vaccine in India: A new framework for vaccine development. Lancet 2014; 383: 2106–2107.

4. Marckwick AJ, Rennels MB, Zito ET, Wade MS, Mack ME. Oral tetravalent rotavirus vaccine can be successfully co-administered with oral polio vaccine and a combined diphtheria, tetanus, pertussis and Haemophilus influenza type B vaccine. US Rhesus Rotavirus Vaccine Study Group. Pediatr Infect Dis J 1998; 17: 913–18.

Chapter 40: Early-life vitamin A supplementation
Dr Robert Dinwiddie, Dr Rob Primhak

(40)

Study: Efficacy of early neonatal supplementation with vitamin A to reduce mortality in infancy in Haryana, India.

Methods: Over a 2-year period, all babies of women aged 15 to 49 were identified in 2 districts of Haryana, India. Eligible participants in a trial of early vitamin A supplementation included those who were able to feed orally and likely to stay in the study area until at least of 6 months of age. Participants were randomly assigned (in blocks of 20) to receive oral vitamin A (50,000 IU) plus vitamin E (9.5–12.6 IU) or placebo-vitamin E (9.5–12.6 IU) within 72 hours of birth.

Parents and researchers were blinded to the treatment given. The primary outcome was mortality between supplementation and 6 months of age. Secondary outcomes were mortality at 12 months of age and reported complications of the treatment.

Findings: 47,777 suitable infants were screened and 44,984 took part in the study. 22,493 received vitamin A and 22,491 placebo. Between supplementation and 6 months of age, 656 infants died in the vitamin A group, compared to 726 in the placebo group (29.2 per 1,000 versus 32.3 per 1,000; difference -3.1 per 1,000 (95% confidence intervals (CI) -6.3 to 0.1, risk ratio 0.90 (95% CI 0.81 to 1.00). At the age of 12 months, 879 infants in the vitamin A group had died compared to 939 in the placebo group (39.1 per 1,000 versus 41.8 per 1,000; difference -2.7 per 1,000 (95% CI -6.3 to 1.00), risk ratio 0.94 (95% CI 0.86 to 1.02).

Vitamin A was generally well tolerated. The incidence of transient bulging fontanelle was 205 in the vitamin A group versus 80 cases in the placebo group, risk ratio 2.56 (95% CI 1.98 to 3.32). Among mothers of the study infants aged 3 months, 39% had low vitamin A status (serum retinol less than 1.05 μmol/l) and 12% had evidence of vitamin A deficiency (serum retinol less than 0.70 μmol/l).

Adapted from Lancet 2015; 385: 1268–71.

Q1. Based on the information shown in the abstract above, which of the following statements is true?

Select <u>one</u> answer only

A. The dropout rate of those eligible versus those studied (6%) reduces the validity of the outcome
B. There was a significant difference in the incidence of transient bulging fontanelle between the treated and the placebo groups
C. There was a significantly higher prevalence of vitamin A deficiency in the mothers of the treated group versus those in the placebo group
D. There was a significantly reduced mortality in the vitamin A supplemented group at 6 months of age
E. There was an excess mortality in the placebo group at the age of 12 months

Q2. Based on a general understanding of the role of vitamin A in infants, which of the following statements regarding trials of supplementation is true?

Select <u>one</u> answer only

A. A double-blind randomised crossover trial would have been a better way to test the effects of vitamin A in this type of population
B. Maternal vitamin A supplementation in pregnancy reduces neonatal mortality
C. The baseline mortality rates in infants studied in different countries are likely to affect the results
D. Vitamin A (50,000 IU) given in the first 72 hours of life is sufficient to maintain adequate serum levels for the first 6 months of life
E. Vitamin A supplementation should be given to all neonates in developing countries

Answers and Rationale

Q1. **B: There was a significant difference in the incidence of transient bulging fontanelle between the treated and the placebo groups**

Q2. **C: The baseline mortality rates in infants studied in different countries are likely to affect the results**

Based on the data shown in the abstract, the dropout rate of 6% is unlikely to affect the results, as the size of the population studied comprised 44,984 individuals. The risk ratio of transient bulging fontanelle was significant in the treated group, 2.56 (95% CI 1.98 to 3.32). If a risk is significant, the confidence intervals of a risk ratio should not include 1, and the confidence intervals for a difference should not include 0. The result for transient bulging fontanelle in this study has a p value of <0.0001, confirming a highly significant difference. The causes and implications of this complication (if any) are still unclear. It is not possible to conclude that there was a significantly higher prevalence of vitamin A deficiency in the mothers of the treated group because the data presented is for both groups of mothers and is not broken down between treated and placebo groups. The mortality rate in the treated group, although showing a modest reduction at 6 months of age, was not quite statistically significant p = 0.056. At 12 months, the risk ratio was 0.94 (95% CI 0.86 to 1.02). In this case, the risk ratio confidence interval includes 1, and the p value is 0.151, which does not reach statistical significance (1, 2).

A double-blind randomised placebo-controlled cross-over trial would not be appropriate due to the fact that there would have to be a washout period between treatments, and it would not be possible to have an uninterrupted follow-up at 6 months of age (3). Maternal vitamin A level supplementation during pregnancy has been shown to not reduce mortality in the neonatal period (4). The baseline mortality rate in any proposed study population is likely to affect the possible results. Parallel studies to this one were carried out in Ghana (5) and Tanzania (6) and clearly did not show any significant effect, probably due to the lower baseline infant mortality rates in those countries. The baseline mortality per 1,000 births in Ghana was 21.8, in Tanzania 24.0, versus 32.3 in India. These factors demonstrate the importance of knowing the baseline population characteristics when designing large studies such as these. Vitamin A at this dose of 50,000 IU showed an increase in vitamin A levels at 2 weeks of age but which was not sustained at 3 months (1, 5, 6). As already noted, the benefits of neonatal vitamin A supplementation in other developing countries were not significant, so it cannot be recommended for widespread use in this age group.

This is an example of a double-blind placebo-controlled trial (3) where 1 group is given a new treatment and compared to a placebo group given an inactive treatment. This is described as a 'negative control' type of study, as opposed to a study where the treated group is compared to a control group given a previously proven treatment (which is a 'positive control' type of study). When designing placebo-controlled trials such as this, it is important to determine in advance the single most important outcome measure, the 'primary outcome'. This is a measure likely to maximise the probability that a positive outcome will change day-to-day clinical practice. Other outcomes ('secondary outcomes') can also be identified, but should be reported separately. This study is an excellent example of one in which the primary outcome was clearly identified as the mortality rate at 6 months of age, with secondary outcomes including the mortality rate at 12 months and side effects such as transient bulging fontanelle being independently analysed. The results presented as the risk ratio of one group compared to another with 95% confidence intervals give an estimate of the range of uncertainty of the results at a 5% level of significance. In general terms, the larger the population studied, the smaller the 95% confidence interval will be. If the confidence intervals include 1.0, then the null hypothesis of the study is rejected.

This was a study sponsored by Bill and Melinda Gates and WHO, from which important messages are to be gained from both the primary and secondary outcome results. The mortality outcome at 6 months is the nearest answer yet to an ongoing debate as to whether or not vitamin A supplementation should be given to infants in the developing Asian countries at birth (1, 2). It further confirms previous studies, which did not show a reduced mortality 12 months. The increased incidence of transient bulging fontanelle also confirms that seen in other studies.

Syllabus Mapping

Science of Practice

- Be able to interpret a research paper or systematic review appropriately

References and Further Reading

1. Mazumba S, Taneja S, Bhatia K, Yoshida S, Kaur K, Dube B, Toteja GS, Bahl R, Fontaine O, Martinez J, Bhandari N. Efficacy of neonatal supplementation with vitamin A to reduce mortality in infancy in Haryana, India (Neovita). Lancet 2015; 385:1333–42.

2. Haider BA, Bhutta ZA. Neonatal vitamin A supplementation: time to move on. Lancet 2015; 385: 1268-71.

3. Anderson M. Trial design. In: Royal College of Paediatrics and Child Health. Clinical cases for the MRCPCH Theory and Science. London, 2013: 197–200.

4. McCauley ME, van den Broek N, Dou L, Othman M. Vitamin A supplementation during pregnancy for maternal and neonatal outcomes. Cochrane Database 2015:CD008666.

5. Edmond KM, Newton S, Shannon C, O'Leary M, Hurt L, Thomas G, Amengo-Etego S, Tawiah-Agyemang C, Gram L, Hurt CN, Bahl R, Owusu-Agyei S, Kirkwood BR. Effect of neonatal vitamin A supplementation on mortality during infancy in Ghana (Neovita): A randomised, double-blind, placebo-controlled trial. Lancet 2015; 385: 1315–23.

6. Masanja H, Smith ER, Mahihi A, Briegleb C, Mshamu S, Ruben J, Noor RA, Khudyakov P, Yoshida S, Martines J, Bahl R, Fawzi WW. Effect of neonatal vitamin A supplementation on mortality in infants in Tanzania (Neovita): A randomised, double-blind, placebo-controlled trial. Lancet 2015; 385: 1342-32.

Chapter 41: A boy with 'fainting' episodes
Dr Robert Dinwiddie and Dr Andrew Boon

(41)

A 14 year old boy presents with episodes of unexpected "collapsing" during sports. He recovers within minutes and appears entirely normal. On examination immediately following an episode, he is fully conscious and alert. There are no heart murmurs but his heart rate is 180/minute. His ECG (taken 1 hour later) is shown below.

Image 41.1: ECG

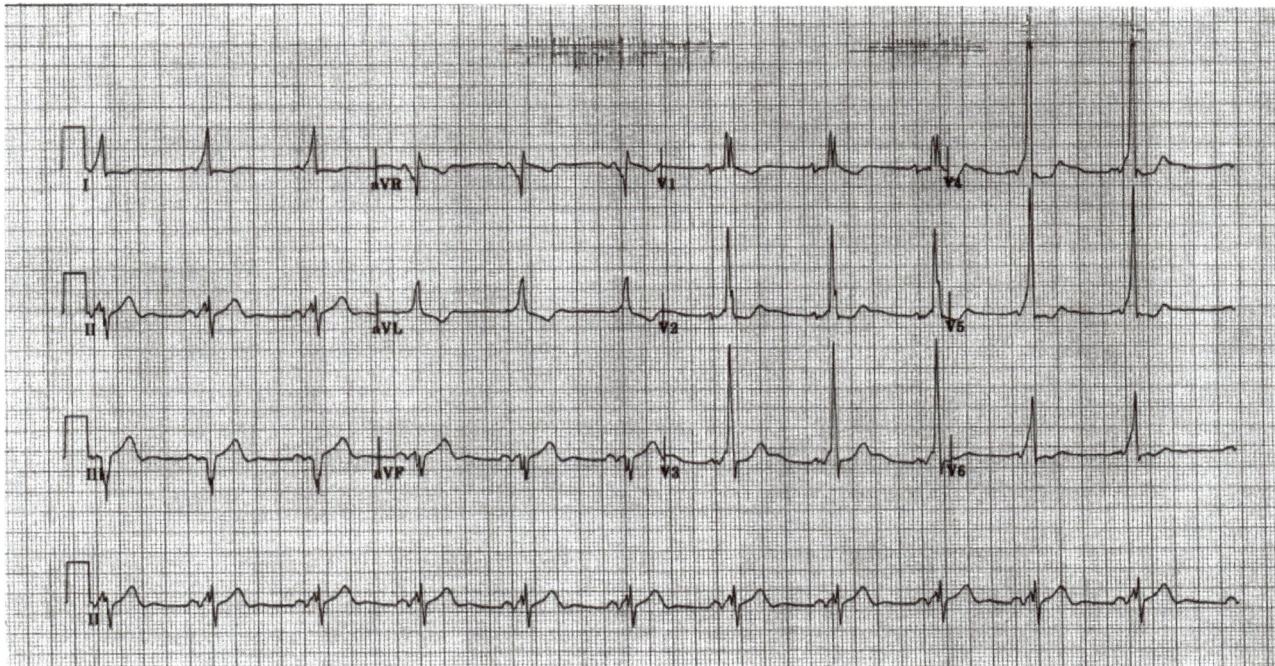

25.0mm/sec   10.0mm/mV

Q1. Which of the following best describes the abnormalities shown on the ECG?

Select one answer only

A. Atrial fibrillation with right bundle branch block
B. Delta waves with first-degree heart block
C. Long QT with atrial ectopics
D. Short PR interval with delta waves
E. Ventricular extrasystoles with sinus bradycardia

Q2. Which of the following is the most likely diagnosis?

Select one answer only

A. Anomalous left coronary artery
B. Atrial septal defect
C. Long QT syndrome
D. Primary pulmonary hypertension
E. Wolff-Parkinson-White syndrome

Answers and Rationale

Q1. **D: Short PR interval with delta waves**
Q2. **E: Wolff-Parkinson-White syndrome**

Delta waves are a slurring of the initial upstroke of the QRS complex. The PR interval in this electrocardiogram (ECG) is 80 milliseconds (two small 1mm squares). The lower limit of normal in the resting ECG at this age is 100 milliseconds (half a larger 5mm square). These are the typical ECG features of Wolff-Parkinson-White (WPW) syndrome. This is a disorder of the cardiac conduction system – one of several cardiac arrhythmias caused by pre-excitation syndromes.

Cardiac arrhythmias in children can result in an increase or decrease in heart rate, and arise due to a number of conditions. These include sinus tachycardia, which rarely exceeds 200 beats/minute, and sinus bradycardia, which can be a consequence of hypoxia, raised intracranial pressure, hypothermia, hypokalaemia, the use of beta-blockers or anorexia. In infants, supraventricular tachycardia (SVT) can present with congestive cardiac failure or circulatory collapse. In older children, SVT can present with palpitations, chest pain or syncope on exertion, as occurred in this case (1).

Other specific cardiac arrhythmias include first-degree heart block. This is demonstrated by a prolonged PR interval on the ECG, and has been associated with conditions such as Lyme disease and rheumatic fever. Second-degree heart block is divided into 2 types – Mobitz type I and Mobitz type II. Mobitz type I results in a prolonged PR interval that steadily increases until a P wave fails to conduct, but is usually asymptomatic. Mobitz type II results in a constant PR interval with random dropping of QRS complexes. Third-degree heart block results in the complete dissociation of atrial and ventricular complexes on the ECG.

The diagnosis, in this case, is WPW syndrome, which is caused by an abnormal electrical conduction pathway between the atria and the ventricles – known as the bundle of Kent. It is thought to be present in approximately 1 in 500 people. If this pathway connects directly from the left atrium to the left ventricle, it can bypass the AV node. The signals passing down this pathway can then result in premature ventricular contractility, resulting in supraventricular tachycardia (SVT) (2).

The normal heartbeat originates as an electrical signal in the sinoatrial node, which is located in the right atrium adjacent to the entry of the superior vena cava. The electrical stimulus then passes through the bundle of His to the right and left bundle branches and, finally, via the Purkinje fibres to the endocardium. Normal heart rate is under the control of the sympathetic and parasympathetic nervous systems through the cardiac control centre in the medulla oblongata. Afferent signals reflecting blood pressure arise in baroreceptors located in the aortic arch. These are transmitted via the vagus nerve to the medulla. Further afferent input occurs through carotid arch stretch receptors via the glossopharyngeal nerves. If the blood pressure is too high, the cardiac control centre then sends efferent signals to the sinoatrial node via the parasympathetic nerve fibres located in the vagus nerve. If the blood pressure is too low, then the cardiac centre delivers efferent signals via the sympathetic nervous system to the sinoatrial/AV node to increase heart rate. In a normal situation, the AV node controls the PR interval, thus preventing the development of an excessive heart rate. This is measured by the PR interval on the ECG, which is normally around 120 milliseconds. With WPW syndrome, this is shortened to less than 100 milliseconds. There is broadening of the QRS complex to greater than 120 milliseconds (90–110 milliseconds is normal in teenagers), typically showing delta waves (3).

The majority of cases of WPW syndrome are sporadic, but a small minority are associated with a positive family history. This syndrome is inherited as an autosomal dominant and is due to a mutation in the *PRKAG2* gene on chromosome 7. Many children with WPW syndrome are asymptomatic. The most frequent clinical presentations are with episodes of dizziness, palpitations and breathlessness. Other clinical features include 'blackouts' and 'fainting' episodes, but cardiac arrest and sudden death is rare (<0.6%).

Treatment of acute episodes is with anti-arrhythmic drugs. When acute episodes are recurrent, then radiofrequency ablation is performed. This is a procedure where a catheter is inserted intravenously into the heart and is targeted towards the possible area of abnormal activity. The area is then mapped electrophysiologically to specifically locate the area of abnormal electrical activity. This area is obliterated by the application of heat radiofrequency ablation or extreme cold (cryo-ablation) from high-frequency radio waves.

Syllabus Mapping

Cardiology

- Be able to assess, diagnose and manage murmurs, chest pain, palpitations, cardiac arrhythmias and syncope.

- Understand investigation of cardiac disease e.g. ECG, ECHO, catheterisation and their appropriate selection in diagnosis and management.

References and Further Reading

1. Price A, Kaski J. How to use the paediatric ECG. Arch Dis Ch Educ Pract Ed 2014; 99: 53–60.

2. Gardiner M, Eisen S, Murphy C. Cardiomyopathy and arrhythmias. In: Gardiner M, Eisen S, Murphy C (eds). Training in Paediatrics. Oxford University Press: Oxford, 2009:90-91.

3. Dickinson DF. The normal ECG in childhood and adolescence. Heart 2005; 91: 1626–1630.

Chapter 42: A 5 year old boy with a rash
Dr Robert Dinwiddie

42

A 5 year old boy is referred to the outpatient clinic because his parents are very concerned about a skin rash involving an increasing number of enlarging and proliferating 'spots' on his arms and trunk. Some have become red and inflamed (see Figure 42.1 below).

Image 42.1

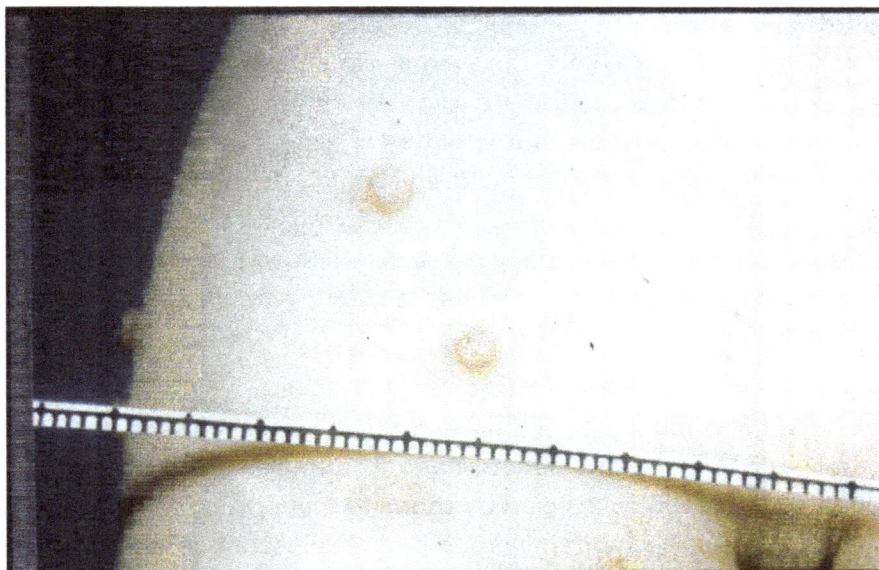

Q1. Which of the following is the best advice to give?

Select <u>one</u> answer only

A.   This appearance may be associated with developmental delay and epilepsy, and needs further investigation
B.   The rash is likely to come and go over several weeks
C.   This is caused by mites and requires not only your child, but all of the family to receive topical treatment
D.   The rash is evidence of an immune deficiency, which will require further investigation
E.   It is due to a bacterial infection that will respond to a course of antibiotics

Q2. Which of the following management options is most appropriate at this stage?

Select <u>one</u> answer only

A.   Application of topical antibiotic cream
B.   Application of topical steroids
C.   Cryotherapy
D.   Observation and reassurance that the lesions will disappear spontaneously
E.   Pulsed laser therapy

Answers and Rationale

Q1. **B: The rash is likely to come and go over several weeks**
Q2. **D: Observation and reassurance that the rash will disappear spontaneously**

The lesions shown in the clinical photograph are typical of molluscum contagiosum. This is a viral infection caused by a DNA pox virus, but one that is not related to the chickenpox or smallpox viruses. All ages can be affected, but it most commonly occurs in children aged 2–5 years. The lesions on the skin are usually multiple and particularly affect the arms, legs and trunk (including the genital areas) but are unusual on the hands and feet. They occasionally affect the eyelids, resulting in follicular conjunctivitis. The incubation period is between 2 and 7 weeks. New lesions can occur while earlier ones are receding. This process can continue over many months and lesions can continue to develop for 12 to 18 months and, occasionally, much longer. The lesions are pinkish white in colour, nodular in appearance and vary from 2 to 9 mm in diameter. A central depression and umbilication are frequent features (1). The infection does not cause any systemic symptoms. Infectivity is low grade, but infection is spread by direct contact and also through the use of shared toys and play objects. Affected children should not share towels, clothing or baths with unaffected siblings. There is, however, no need to avoid gymnastics or swimming at school (2). In adolescents and adults, the infection can be sexually transmitted. Secondary eczema can develop around the lesions, especially in atopic individuals. The associated eczema increases itchiness and scratching, which may spread the lesions further.

The lesions shown in the figure are not typical of adenoma sebaceum, such as would be seen in tuberous sclerosis. Thus, they would not be associated with impaired intellect or need further neurological investigation. They are not typical in appearance for scabies, caused by the mite *Sarcoptes scabiei*, so would not need topical therapy either for the patient or other family members. Molluscum contagiosum is commonly more severe in the immunocompromised, especially those with HIV infection, but this is not usually the first presentation of these conditions. Because it is a viral infection, antibiotics are not indicated unless there is secondary bacterial infection of individual lesions, when fusidic acid may be useful. Topical steroids such as hydrocortisone cream can be used with emollients in atopic individuals when itching is severe.

Specific treatment is not indicated, as the lesions heal spontaneously after several weeks or months. Parents should be reassured that watchful waiting is the best approach. If there is infection of the eyelids, then urgent referral to ophthalmology is indicated. Infectivity to others is low especially if scratching is avoided by keeping the fingernails short. In some cases, however, the lesions do cause troublesome symptoms. Treatment options in these situations include physical puncture of individual lesions and the removal of the contents. This can be painful, so it is recommended that local anaesthetic is used in advance of the treatment. The fluid contents are infectious, so there is a risk of local spreading. Cryotherapy, in which liquid nitrogen is applied to individual lesions for 5 to 10 seconds, is effective after the application of local anaesthetic. Pulsed laser therapy is utilised in some specialist dermatology clinics. Other agents that are used in specialist clinics include podophyllotoxin (which can, however, be irritant), imiquimod and cidofovir, although there is no clinical trial evidence of specific efficacy for this condition. If lesions are left to resolve spontaneously, scarring is rare but it is more likely to occur if direct therapy is used. Immunity following an episode is usually lifelong and recurrence is rare.

Syllabus Mapping

Dermatology

• Be able to assess, diagnose and manage skin infections in children

References and Further Reading

1. Jones C, Isaacs D. Miscellaneous viral infections. In: McIntosh N, Helms P, Smyth R, Logan S (eds). Forfar and Arneil's Textbook of Paediatrics, 7th edition. Churchill Livingstone Elsevier: Edinburgh, 2008: 1300–1302.

2. http://cks.nice.org.uk/molluscum-contagiosum September 2012.

Chapter 43: A newborn baby with floppiness
Professor Win Tin, Dr Ramesh Kumar

(43)

A male infant with a birthweight of 3.5 kg was admitted from the postnatal ward to the neonatal unit at about 10 hours of age with a history of poor feeding, lethargy and floppiness. He was born by normal delivery at term, and was noted to have the umbilical cord around his neck. He received inflation breaths due to poor respiratory effort at birth, but did not need any further resuscitation. He is the first child of non-consanguineous parents. There are no antenatal concerns and the maternal medical history is unremarkable. Cord blood pH is 7.2 with base excess of -7.3.

On examination at the time of admission, his temperature is 37.3°C, and he is well perfused with oxygen saturations of 97% in air. Examination of his cardiovascular system, respiratory system and abdomen do not show any abnormalities. He is noted to have generalised hypotonia and paucity of spontaneous body movements. There are no dysmorphic features, and his head circumference and length are on the 50th centiles. His external genitalia appear normal. His blood glucose on admission was 4.2 mmol/l. He is started on intravenous antibiotics after the blood culture was taken.

Investigations

Blood

Haemoglobin	160 g/l
White cell count	11.2 x 10⁹/l
Platelets	250 x 10⁹/l
Urea	4.2 mmol/l
Sodium	136 mmol/
Potassium	3.7 mmol/l
Creatinine	52 μmol/l
Calcium	2.2 mmol/l
Magnesium	0.9 mmol/l
CRP	<5 mg/dl

He is noted as having frequent and profound apnoeic episodes since about 6 hours after his admission, and requires mechanical ventilation. He is also noted as having intermittent hiccups and myoclonic jerking movements of all limbs while he is on the ventilator.

Q1. What is the most likely diagnosis?

Select one answer only

A.   Congenital myotonic dystrophy
B.   Hypoxic-ischaemic encephalopathy (HIE) (grade 3)
C.   Non-ketotic hyperglycinaemia (glycine encephalopathy)
D.   Prader-Willi syndrome
E.   Spinal muscular atrophy type 1 (Werdnig-Hoffmann disease)

Q2. Name the investigation most likely to confirm the diagnosis.

Select one answer only

A.   Amplitude-integrated electroencephalogram (EEG)
B.   FISH for detection of 15q11.2
C.   Molecular genetic testing for cytosine-thymine-guanine (CTG) expansion of DMPK gene
D.   Molecular genetic testing for homozygous deletions of axon 7 and 8 of SMN1 gence
E.   Plasma and CSF glycine (paired sample)

Answers and Rationale

Q1. **C: Non-ketotic hyperglycinaemia (glycine encephalopathy)**
Q2. **E: Plasma and CSF glycine (paired sample)**

Non-ketotic hyperglycinaemia, also known as glycine encephalopathy (GCE), is an autosomal recessive inborn error of glycine degradation that leads to excessive accumulation of glycine in all tissues, particularly in the central nervous system (1). The underlying defect is a deficiency of the glycine cleavage system (GCS), an intra-mitochondrial enzyme complex made up of 4 different protein components.

Glycine functions both as an inhibitory and excitatory neurotransmitter. GCS deficiency causes an accumulation of glycine in the synaptic cleft, leading to an overstimulation of the N-methyl-D-aspartate (NMDA) receptor. This causes an increased intracellular free calcium accumulation, resulting in neuronal injury, with subsequent cell death and intractable seizures. Glycine is an inhibitory neurotransmitter on glycinergic receptors, located in the spinal cord and the brain stem. Stimulation results in increased permeability to chloride in the post-synaptic neurons and is likely to be involved in muscular hypotonia, neonatal apnoea and hiccups.

The prevalence of non-ketotic hyperglycinaemia is approximately 1 in 60,000. Most newborns with the severe form (classical non-ketotic hyperglycinaemia) present within the first 2 days of life with hypotonia, hiccups, multi-focal myoclonus, seizures, stupor and coma. Hiccups are a particularly helpful clinical sign.

Most infants with the classic form die (over 50% in the first week), and survivors have severe developmental disabilities. Patients with the milder form show variable degrees of learning difficulties, epilepsy, behavioural problems and movement disorders. Patients with the transient form are rare but with a better neurological outcome. Non-ketotic hyperglycinaemia is diagnosed biochemically by the typical combination of an increase of glycine in the plasma and CSF, with an increased CSF to plasma glycine ratio that is pathognomonic of this condition.

There is currently no effective treatment for non-ketotic hyperglycinaemia, and cessation of life support is often considered due to the very poor prognosis.

Other causes of neonatal hypotonia

In newborns with severe HIE, there is usually a history of fetal distress, such as reduced fetal movements or meconium stained liquor, requirement of resuscitation, low cord pH and the features of other major organ dysfunction, in addition to early onset encephalopathy. Mostly, features of encephalopathy are present soon after birth, but the presentation may be delayed sometimes. The presence of hiccups is not a typical feature of HIE.

Amplitude integrated EEG is a useful monitoring tool in newborns with HIE for the assessment of the severity of encephalopathy, the selection of patients for neuroprotective intervention, the detection of seizures, the evaluation of the effect of anticonvulsants and the prediction of neurodevelopmental outcome.

Prader-Willi Syndrome can present in the neonatal period, its common features being hypotonia, poor feeding, characteristic craniofacial features (dolichocephaly, almond-shaped eyes, small appearing mouth and the upper lips) and hypogonadism. Respiratory difficulty that requires ventilator support is uncommon, and hiccups are not a feature of Prader-Willi syndrome. The mainstay of diagnosis is genetic testing (detection of 15q11.2 by FISH).

The infants with congenital myotonic dystrophy are born to mothers often with a history of polyhydramnios and reduced fetal movements. The infants have significant hypotonia (rather than myotonia, as in adult patients) with muscle weakness, especially their facial muscles in most cases. Many infants also present with club feet and facial dysmorphism. The respiratory insufficiency presents early, so that the baby needs ventilator support soon after birth. Hiccups are not a clinical feature.

Congenital myotonic dystrophy is caused by an unstable trinucleotide repeat expansion containing CTG in the DMPK (DM1) gene located at chromosome region 19q13.3, and the DNA-based testing is now available to diagnose this condition.

Infants with spinal muscular atrophy type 1 (Werdnig-Hoffmann disease) present with profound weakness and hypotonia, but with relatively preserved facial movements. Contractures at wrists and ankles are evident at birth in some infants. Most newborns will have a bell-shaped chest, paradoxical chest movement and intercostal recession. Diagnosis can be made based on a muscle biopsy, but a specific DNA test (for homozygous deletions of axon 7 and 8 of SMN1 gene) is also available.

Syllabus Mapping

Neonatology

- Be able to assess, diagnose and manage neurological disorders and make appropriate referral

Neurology

- Be able to assess, diagnose and manage seizure disorders and conditions which may mimic them

Reference

1. Hennermann J. Clinical variability in glycine encephalopathy. Future Neurol 2006; 1(5): 621–630.

Further Reading

Volpe JJ. Neurology of the Newborn, 5th edition. WB Saunders: Philadelphia, 2008.

Rennie JM. Rennie and Roberton's Textbook of Neonatology, 5th edition. Churchill Livingstone: Elsevier Ltd, 2012.

Chapter 44: A boy with early puberty
Dr Joanna Walker

An 8 year old boy is referred to a paediatric outpatient clinic with concerns about sexual precocity. He has had adult sweat odour for 2–3 years and his parents think his penis is larger than it should be. He also has some pubic hair and acne. On examination, he is a generally healthy boy. His height is on the 91st centile compared with a mid-parental centile of the 50th. His weight is on the 75th. He has moderate facial acne. The testicular volumes are 8 ml bilaterally, and he has reached Tanner Stage 3 for genital and pubic hair development. The remainder of the examination is normal.

Q1. Which of the following is the most likely diagnosis?

Select <u>one</u> answer only

A.   Adrenal carcinoma
B.   Congenital adrenal hyperplasia
C.   Craniopharyngioma
D.   Hypothalamic hamartoma
E.   Normal early puberty

Q2. Which of the following will confirm the diagnosis?

Select <u>one</u> answer only

A.   Abdominal ultrasound scan
B.   Bone age estimation
C.   Cranial magnetic resonance imaging (MRI) scan
D.   Serum testosterone
E.   Urine steroid profile

Answer and Rationale

Q1.   D: Hypothalamic hamartoma
Q2.   C: Cranial magnetic resonance imaging (MRI) scan

Answering this question requires knowledge of normal pubertal development. Puberty should only start from the age of 8 years in a girl and 9 years in a boy. In both sexes, it follows a set *tempo*, staged clinically using the Tanner criteria (1). In girls, there is gradual breast and pubic hair development with the peak velocity of the growth spurt at mid-puberty. Menarche comes towards the end of puberty, when growth is already slowing. In boys, there is gradual enlargement of the testes, development of pubic hair and secondary sexual characteristics. The peak height velocity is higher in boys and reached later than in girls because higher concentrations of testosterone are needed to maximise growth compared with oestrogen. Thus, on average, men are taller than women. Shaving marks the final steps of male puberty. It is important to know these stages or where to find details.

However, many girls will start normal puberty earlier and pathology is rare. It is often related to excess weight and family history, and is also more common in girls from certain racial backgrounds. It might therefore still need managing if socially unacceptable at such a young age. Puberty may be abnormally early in girls with developmental problems, such as cerebral palsy and neurometabolic conditions. In boys, significant pathology is much more likely and early puberty should always be investigated.

When assessing early puberty – sexual precocity – we use the history and examination to determine what hormone(s) must be responsible and then consider the possible sources and relevant investigations. The causes are best considered to be gonadotrophin dependent or independent. The former will include children, like this boy, who are developing at a normal tempo but are too young, so the answer is not normal puberty. His enlarging testes are clinical evidence of the activation of the hypothalamic-pituitary-testicular axis, excluding adrenal carcinoma or congenital adrenal hyperplasia as diagnoses. He is tall for family size and this is not related to him being overweight, which is usually the most common cause for being tall for family during childhood. A cranial MRI scan is mandatory. A hypothalamic hamartoma (tuber cinereum hamartoma) is found in 33% of cases. Lack of enhancement with contrast media helps distinguish it from rarer causes such as a germ cell tumour or Langerhans cell histiocytosis.

Other tumours in this location, such as craniopharyngioma, usually present with evidence of pituitary hormone deficiency (particularly growth failure due to growth hormone deficiency) or raised intracranial pressure. Hypothalamic hamartoma are benign congenital tumours and best left alone unless associated with gelastic (laughter) seizures that are resistant to drug treatment, in which case, specialist surgical techniques may be considered. Gonadotrophin-dependent sexual precocity in either sex due to a pathological cause or where it is deemed socially undesirable is managed – usually very successfully – with a gonadotrophin-releasing hormone analogue.

Gonadotrophin-independent sexual precocity describes children who have evidence of hormone production but the tempo is abnormal. For example, a 2 year old girl with breast development – i.e.

premature thelarche. The hormone responsible must be oestrogen. This is common and usually benign, as evidenced by the lack of growth acceleration and other secondary sexual characteristics, particularly 'oestrogenisation' of the external genitalia. It tends to regress over time and is ill-understood.

The most common cause of gonadotrophin-independent sexual precocity is exaggerated adrenarche. Adrenarche is a normal event in all children when, roughly between the ages of 5 and 8 years, the zona reticularis of the adrenal cortex matures and starts to produce some mild androgens. These are probably responsible for a mid-childhood growth spurt but, otherwise, usually go unnoticed. However, some children develop adult sweat odour ± acne ± pubic hair. The latter is characteristically long and sparse and confined to the labia in girls and the base of the penis in boys. A pathological source of androgens is excluded by the absence of other evidence of virilisation – e.g. growth acceleration, clitoromegaly, and secondary sexual characteristics.

Elevated testosterone is the best, albeit non-specific, biochemical marker of excess androgen irrespective of the source. Exaggerated adrenarche used to be considered a benign event, but is now known to be linked to insulin resistance and thereby the risk of metabolic syndrome in adulthood. It is most common in overweight girls, and their families should be counselled about this risk and offered support in the management of their daughter's weight.

The likeliest pathological cause of gonadotrophin-independent sexual precocity will be congenital adrenal hyperplasia, which can be excluded with a urine steroid profile. Adrenal carcinoma is rare and usually visible on an abdominal ultrasound.

Syllabus Mapping

Endocrinology and Growth

* Know the causes of problems relating to growth and puberty. Be able to assess, diagnose and manage, referring when appropriate

Reference and Further Reading

1. Raine JE, Donaldson MDC, Gregory J, Van-Vliet G. Practical Endocrinology and Diabetes in Children, 3rd edition. Wiley-Blackwell, 2011. ISBN: 978-1-4051-9634-5.

Chapter 45: A 10 year old girl passing 'dark urine'
Dr Fiona Hickey, Dr Simone Stokley

45

A 10 year old girl is admitted while on her summer holiday with a 6-hour history of passing 'dark urine'. She is otherwise well but had recently been started on antibiotics for a presumed urinary tract infection (UTI). She has had ligation of a patent arterial duct (ductus arteriosus) at the age of 8 months, and had been diagnosed with complex partial seizures 12 months before this admission. She was on carbamazepine for her seizures and had been fit-free since starting treatment. The patient was born in the UK to parents from the Mediterranean area.

On examination, she is pale and has several small lymph nodes palpable in the cervical chain but is otherwise generally well. Heart sounds and blood pressure are normal. There are no abnormalities on examination of the cardiovascular, respiratory and abdominal systems.

Investigations

Blood

Haemoglobin	82 g/l
MCV	90 fl (75–87)
MCH	29 pg (25–37)
MCHC	310 g/dl (32–35)
White cell count	5.2 x 10^9/l
Platelets	460 x 10^9/l
Reticulocytes	362 x 10^9/l
Coombs test	negative
Ferritin	28 µg/l (12–200)
B$_{12}$	314 ng/l (160–925)

Q1. Which investigation is the most likely to lead to the explanation of the dark urine?

Select <u>one</u> answer only

A.   Bone marrow aspirate and trephine
B.   Cold agglutinins
C.   EMA binding test
D.   G6PD assay
E.   Haemoglobin electrophoresis

Q2. What is the next appropriate step in management?

Select <u>one</u> answer only

A.   Arrange plasmapheresis
B.   Give IV methylprednisolone
C.   Repeat FBC in 1 hour
D.   Start oral prednisolone
E.   Transfuse red blood cells

Answers and Rationale

Q1. **D: G6PD assay**
Q2. **C: repeat FBC in 1 hour**

A child presenting with a sudden onset of dark urine and anaemia is highly suggestive of acute haemolysis. Clinical jaundice and a raised unconjugated bilirubin would add to this diagnosis. Red blood cell indices indicate normocytic, normochromic anaemia and a raised reticulocyte count (and therefore a marrow capable of responding to the haemolysis). The Mediterranean connection may raise the possibility of thalassaemia, but one would expect microcytic, hypochromic anaemia. Cardiac valve surgery and some anticonvulsants can produce similar symptoms but the timing of the events make those unlikely. The recent prescription of antibiotics – possibly nitrofurantoin – suggests that this is the precipitating cause in a child with undiagnosed G6PD deficiency (1). The EMA binding test looks for spherocytosis.

The offending precipitating antibiotics will be stopped while the diagnosis is confirmed. The red blood cell haemolysis should then slow. It is important to establish the rate of fall of the red blood cells, and hence the need to repeat the FBC after an interval. Red blood cell transfusion would only be necessary when the patient becomes symptomatic and it may be possible to avoid transfusion completely.

The definition of anaemia changes with age and ranges from values below 110 g/l in children between 6 and 60 months, below 115 g/l in children up to 11 years of age, and below 120 g/l in young adolescents. The World Health Organization (WHO) also provides a definition of severe anaemia that is below 70 g/l for those under 5 years and below 80 g/l for older children and adolescents (2, 3).

Anaemia is very common in early childhood and is usually the result of insufficient iron within the diet. This age group also has a high consumption of cow's milk, which is a poor source of iron. Studies and surveys have demonstrated that up to 3% of children under the age of 24 months are anaemic, but this varies widely. Some ethnic groups in the UK and children in low-income families have a much higher incidence.

It is important to clarify whether the anaemia is an isolated finding or whether it is part of a pancytopaenia. If the latter, then causes of marrow failure should be explored and bone marrow aspirate and trephine are usually required.

An isolated anaemia can be viewed as the result of a problem with the production, or an excessive loss or increased destruction of red blood cells.

The history and an examination will offer direction to the underlying diagnosis, but the red blood cell indices will provide further information. The mean corpuscular volume (MCV) provides a structured way to categorise anaemia, with cells being microcytic, normocytic or macrocytic.

Microcytic anaemia is most commonly the result of an inadequate uptake of iron – either from reduced amounts within the diet or poor absorption (as seen in coeliac disease). In the absence of other features in the history or on examination, and in the presence of a low ferritin, the diagnosis is that of iron deficiency and management would be with a trial of oral iron supplementation.

A family history of anaemia, or Mediterranean, Asian or African ethnicity should prompt the consideration of alpha or beta thalassaemia. In these conditions, there is a problem with the alpha or beta haemoglobin chain production. Carriers of beta thalassaemia (beta thalassaemia trait) have raised levels of HbA2 and HbF (1).

The anaemia of chronic illness is usually hypochromic, and can be either microcytic or normocytic, but the mechanism is not well understood. It is likely due to the dysregulation of iron homeostasis with macrophages taking up iron along with an impaired proliferation of erythroid cells due to cytokines. There may also be an inadequate response to erythropoietin (4).

A normocytic anaemia can be the result of blood loss or haemolysis. Where there is an excess loss – such as in acute haemolysis – a normal marrow will generate immature red blood cells, leading to a rise in the circulating reticulocyte count. It then becomes necessary to identify the cause of haemolysis, which could be a membrane abnormality (spherocytosis), an absence of a red blood cell enzyme (G6PD deficiency, pyruvate kinase) or haemoglobinopathy (sickle cell, thalassaemia). An autoimmune haemolytic anaemia (primary or secondary to a range of conditions) or microangiopathic haemolytic anaemia (HUS, DIC, TTP) will also produce a normocytic anaemia.

A reduced reticulocyte count indicates that the marrow is unable to respond to the increased demand, as seen with responses to some infections and certain drugs.

It is also useful to consider the nutritional status of the patient and measure other haematinics, as an early vitamin B_{12} or folate deficiency or an iron deficiency with concurrent vitamin B_{12} or folate deficiency could present with a normal MCV. Where there is no evidence of the above conditions and in the setting of a severe or persistent anaemia, it may be necessary to perform a bone marrow aspirate and trephine.

A macrocytic anaemia can be due to vitamin B_{12} or folate deficiency, although these conditions are very rare in childhood. A careful drug history may reveal drugs that can interfere with the folate metabolism, such as methotrexate (a dihydrofolate reductase inhibitor). A haemolytic anaemia will lead to an increase in reticulocyte production and, as these are large cells, the measured MCV will show a macrocytosis, as in the present case.

Macrocytosis can also be seen in patients with congenital heart disease, Down syndrome, hypothyroidism, liver disease, and asplenia, and with certain drugs. However, the anaemia in these patients is usually very mild. In the case of a macrocytic anaemia with no identified cause, a bone marrow may be indicated, as this could identify a rare cause such as Diamond-Blackfan anaemia or Fanconi anaemia.

Syllabus Mapping

Haematology and Oncology

- Be able to assess, diagnose and manage children with anaemia including bone marrow failure and know when to refer

References and Further Reading

1. Cappellini MD, Fiorelli G. Glucose-6-phosphate dehydrogenase deficiency . Lancet 2008; 371: 64-74.

2. World Health Organisation. Haemoglobin concentrations for the diagnosis of anaemia and assessment of severity. Geneva, 2011.

3. Booth IW, Aukett MA. Iron deficiency anaemia in infancy and early childhood. Archives of disease in childhood 1997; 76: 549-554.

4. Weiss G, Goodnough LT. Anemia of chronic disease. New England Journal of Medicine 2005; 352: 1011-1023.

Chapter 46: A child with abdominal pain
Dr Rob Primhak

A 3 year old boy presents to your clinic with a 1 year history of abdominal pain, with periods of constipation, alternating with periods of loose stools. He is reported to pass a hard stool once weekly with difficulty, but also has periods of loose stools for a few days every month with some soiling. He is said to be generally irritable and lethargic. He is a fussy eater, has a poor appetite and does not like vegetables or fruit. He also has had several prolonged episodes of mouth ulcers. He is fractious on examination, but has mild abdominal distension, with no palpable masses. His weight and height are on the 10th centile; his parent-held record shows that he followed the 25th centile for the first 2 years and there were no measurements for the last year.

Blood results

Haemoglobin	109 g/l
White cell count	7.2 x 10⁹/l
MCV	68 fl
MCH	25 pg (27–33)
MCHC	30 g/dl (32–35)
Platelets	540 x 10⁹/l

Q1. What is the most likely diagnosis?

Select one answer only

A. Behçet's disease
B. Coeliac disease
C. Crohn's disease
D. Diet-related constipation with overflow
E. Hirschsprung's disease

Q2. Which of the following investigations would be most helpful at this point?

Select three answers only

A. Anti-tissue transglutaminase antibodies
B. Dietetic assessment
C. Faecal calprotectin
D. HLA haplotype
E. Ileocolonoscopy with biopsy
F. Immunoglobulin A (IgA) level
G. Immunoglobulin G (IgG) and immunoglobulin M (IgM) levels
H. Rectal biopsy
I. Slit lamp examination of eyes
J. Stool culture and faecal occult blood
K. Upper GI endoscopy and duodenal biopsy

Answers and Rationale

Q1.   **B: Coeliac disease**
Q2.   **A: Anti-tissue transglutaminase antibodies**
            B: Dietetic assessment
            F: Immunoglobulin A (IgA) level

The choice of investigations depends on the likely differential diagnosis. This patient has unexplained abdominal symptoms and haematological findings suggestive of iron deficiency. His weight and height velocity appears to have reduced. The most likely diagnosis in this case is coeliac disease. A poor diet that is low in fibre and iron can cause poor weight gain with constipation and overflow, but when seen together with growth impairment and prolonged episodes of aphthous ulcers, organic pathology is likely.

Lethargy and irritability can happen in malnutrition with any cause, but is particularly prominent in coeliac disease. Aphthous ulcers – if short-lived and infrequent – usually do not imply any underlying disease, but frequent and persistent aphthae occur in 16% of children with coeliac disease, 9% of those with Crohn's disease, and rarely in ulcerative colitis. Behçet's disease is uncommon in childhood; the oral ulcers are almost always associated with genital ulcers, rashes, eye symptoms or arthritis, and abdominal symptoms are rare.

Although Hirschsprung's disease usually presents in infancy, it can occasionally present later with constipation, but very rarely causes soiling and the lack of symptoms in the first 2 years makes it very unlikely.

Once the likely differential diagnosis has been considered, the most important diagnosis to confirm or exclude with this presentation is coeliac disease. The recommended initial test for this is the presence of IgA antibody to tissue transglutaminase. It is essential to exclude IgA deficiency when performing this test, as there is an association between IgA deficiency and coeliac disease, and this combination would yield a false negative result. A dietetic assessment would be appropriate to document adequate intake of gluten, essential before serological testing and to record baseline dietary adequacy. Faecal calprotectin is a useful marker of inflammatory bowel disease, but in children under 4 years it is unreliable (1).

The definitive investigation in the diagnosis of coeliac disease is a duodenal biopsy. Current guidelines do not require a biopsy for confirmation only if the child has a) suggestive symptoms AND b) anti-tissue transglutaminase antibodies >10 times the upper limit of normal AND c) positive anti-endomysial antibodies, AND d) HLA DQ2 or DQ8 positive on testing (2). Nevertheless, many centres would still perform a confirmatory duodenal biopsy if anti-tissue transglutaminase antibodies were present, particularly in the infant or younger child.

Coeliac disease can have a protean presentation. In a series of 263 paediatric patients in New Zealand, diarrhoea was present in only 38%, abdominal pain in 43%, and constipation in 6%. One third had iron deficiency and one quarter had poor weight gain. In children under 5, at presentation, the weight and height z-scores were equivalent at -0.4, and less than 10% of the children were below the 3rd centile for weight at presentation (3).

The incidence of diagnosed coeliac disease has increased over recent years, although it is not clear if there is a genuine increase in incidence or an improvement in diagnostic methods and awareness. Thus, it is important to keep a high index of suspicion for this condition.

About one third of newly diagnosed cases are asymptomatic, and detected by the screening of high-risk populations (4). Screening with HLA testing and IgA anti-tissue transglutaminase is recommended in: type 1 diabetes, Down syndrome, Williams syndrome, Turner syndrome (TS), autoimmune thyroiditis, autoimmune liver disease and unexplained raised transaminases. Appropriate screening is also recommended in children with selective IgA deficiency and first-degree relatives of coeliac patients (2).

Syllabus Mapping

Gastroenterology and Hepatology

- Be able to assess, diagnose and manage conditions resulting in malabsorption including coeliac disease

Reference and Further Reading

1. Hansen R, Russell RK, Muhammed R. Recent advances in paediatric gastroenterology. Arch Dis Child. 2015; 100(9): 886–90.

2. Murch S, Jenkins H, Auth M et al. Joint BSPGHAN and Coeliac UK guidelines for the diagnosis and management of coeliac disease in children. *Arch Dis Child* 2013; 98: 806–811.

3. Kho A, Whitehead M, Day AS. Coeliac disease in children in Christchurch, New Zealand: Presentation and patterns from 2000–2010. *World Journal of Clinical Pediatrics* 2015; 4(4): 148–154.

4. Whyte LA, Jenkins HR. The epidemiology of coeliac disease in South Wales: A 28-year perspective. *Arch Dis Child* 2013; 98(6): 405–407.

Chapter 47: A 14 year old girl with headaches
Dr Robert Dinwiddie

(47)

A 14 year old girl presents with a 3 month history of recurrent headaches. These occur on a daily basis and are worse when lying flat or bending down. Her BMI is 28.8 kg/m². The neurological examination is normal except for a right sixth nerve palsy and evidence of early bilateral papilloedema. Blood pressure is 130/75 mmHg. The MRI brain scan is reported as normal.

Investigations

Blood

	Full blood count	normal
	Glucose	4.5 mmol/l
	Urea and electrolytes	normal

CSF

	Appearance	clear, no red blood cells, no white blood cells
	Protein	0.4 g/l
	Glucose	3.5 mmol/l
	Gram stain	negative
	Opening pressure	30 cm H_2O (23 mmHg)

Q1. Which of the following is the most likely diagnosis?

Select one answer only

A. Hypertensive encephalopathy
B. Idiopathic intracranial hypertension (IIH)
C. Intracranial tumour
D. Migraine
E. Recurrent ingestion of methylenedioxymethamphetamine (ecstasy)

Q2. Which of the following is the most important complication?

Select one answer only

A. Hydrocephalus
B. Intracranial haemorrhage
C. Loss of visual acuity
D. Retinal haemorrhage
E. Stroke

Q3. Which of the following treatment regimens has the best effect in preventing the most important long-term complication at this stage?

Select one answer only

A. Acetazolamide
B. Furosemide
C. IV mannitol
D. Prednisolone
E. Repeat lumbar punctures

Answers and Rationale

Q1. **B: Idiopathic intracranial hypertension (IIH)**
Q2. **C: Loss of visual acuity**
Q3. **A: Acetazolamide**

The clinical history and investigations make IIH the most likely diagnosis. The blood pressure of 130/75 mmHg is at the upper limit of the normal range for a 14 year old girl, making hypertensive encephalopathy unlikely. Recurrent headaches, a sixth nerve palsy and papilloedema could be indicative of an intracranial tumour, but this would frequently be associated with vomiting, especially in the morning. The normal MRI head scan excludes this diagnosis. Migraines have been reported in association with IIH, but papilloedema is not a feature. Recurrent drug abuse, including ecstasy, would result in acute episodic symptoms, which are not a feature in this case.

IIH is, by definition, a diagnosis reached by the exclusion of other causes of increased intracranial pressure. The diagnostic criteria for classic IIH include: the presence of papilloedema, a normal neurological examination (except for cranial nerve abnormalities), normal brain parenchyma without evidence of hydrocephalus, mass, or structural lesions and no abnormal meningeal enhancement on MRI, and MRI venography with and without gadolinium, normal CSF composition but elevated lumbar puncture opening pressure (>25-cm H_2O, or >28-cm H_2O if obese or sedated) in a properly performed lumbar puncture (1,2).

IIH is known to be significantly associated with obesity. The female to male ratio is 2:1. The prevalence of IIH, particularly in adolescence, is increasing as the incidence of obesity in this age group rises. It is therefore important to calculate the BMI and to provide relevant dietary advice as part of overall management. One other important cause of raised intracranial pressure is cerebral venous sinus thrombosis; this would be evident on a venous MRI scan. IIH is also associated with a number of other medical conditions and medications (1). The clinical history and examination should therefore exclude evidence of chronic otitis media, mastoiditis or sinusitis, hypothyroidism and hyperthyroidism, Cushing's disease, adrenal insufficiency, vitamin D deficiency and systemic lupus erythematosus. Drugs associated with the development of IIH include antibiotics (e.g. tetracyclines, sulphonamides, nitrofurantoin and penicillin), hormones (e.g. levothyroxine, growth hormone) and those contained in oral contraceptive pills. Other reported causes include ciclosporin, phenytoin, vitamin A analogues and isotretinoin.

Partial or complete loss of vision occurs in 20–40% of IIH cases, making this the most important long-term complication. Hydrocephalus, intracranial haemorrhage and stroke are known complications of IIH. If hydrocephalus is found, it should prompt a search for other underlying causes of raised intracranial pressure. Retinal haemorrhage has been described in association with IIH, but is not the most important long-term complication.

Close follow-up and treatment is important in order to monitor for early signs of visual loss. This should involve a multidisciplinary team, including the primary paediatrician, ophthalmologist, orthoptist, paediatric neurologist and a neurosurgeon (1). At lumbar puncture, it is recommended that the CSF pressure is reduced to 15–20 cmH$_2$O. Repeat lumbar punctures only provide temporary relief. The most frequently used medication for IIH is acetazolamide, a carbonic anhydrase inhibitor that is thought to act by reducing the volume of CSF produced. It is the most effective treatment for the prevention of long-term complications (1, 3). Furosemide is not the most effective initial treatment but is used in conjunction with acetazolamide in resistant cases. Corticosteroids, such as prednisolone, are not recommended for continuous use, but may be useful as acute additional therapy during crises and in those patients whose vision is threatened while waiting for surgery. Mannitol is also useful but only during acute crises. Various surgical interventions have been used, including ventriculo-peritoneal shunting, lumbo-peritoneal shunting, optic nerve fenestration and, if it is narrowed, endovascular stenting of the transverse sinus.

The majority of patients respond to treatment, and the condition gradually resolves over a period of many months. A minority do, however, develop significant permanent visual loss and have recurrent headaches despite the intensive treatment regimens currently available.

Syllabus Mapping

Neurology

- Know the investigation and management of headache including unusual causes such as raised intracranial pressure

References and Further Reading

1. Babiker MOE, Prasad M, MacLeod S, Chow G, Whitehouse WP. Fifteen-minute consultation: The child with idiopathic intracranial hypertension. Arch Dis Child Educ Pract Ed 2014; 99: 166–172.

2. Avery RA, Shah SS, Licht DJ et al. Reference range for cerebrospinal fluid opening pressure in children. N Engl J Med 2010; 363: 891–893.

3. Matthews YY. Drugs used in childhood idiopathic or benign intracranial hypertension. Arch Dis Child Educ Pract Ed 2008; 93: 19–25.

Chapter 48: A newborn baby with respiratory distress
Dr Shalabh Garg, Dr Ruppa Mohanram Geethanath

48

A baby boy was born at 39 weeks of gestation by normal delivery. The mother had a proven UTI caused by group B Streptococcus 3 weeks before delivery, and received a full course of antibiotics. Thin meconium staining of liquor was noted at birth, but the baby did not require any resuscitation. He was noted to have grunting respiration with a respiratory rate of 60/minute at 2 hours of age. His temperature was 37°C, and his oxygen saturation in air was 95%. He was admitted to the neonatal unit and was commenced on nasal CPAP. He was also commenced on intravenous antibiotics after a blood culture was taken. His chest x-ray (taken at 4 hours of age) is shown (Figure 27.1).

The baby received nasal CPAP for about 48 hours. The C-reactive protein sample taken on day 1 was 5 mg/dl. Antibiotics were stopped on day 3, when the blood culture was reported as negative. He was discharged home on day 6, when his respiratory distress settled and full breastfeeding was established, with a plan to follow up at 6 weeks of age and to repeat a chest x-ray at that stage.

The baby was noted be gaining weight and was reported to be feeding well when reviewed. His parents did not express any concerns but mentioned that he developed a dry cough over the last 2 weeks. He was noted to be tachypnoeic, with intercostal and subcostal recession. His oxygen saturation in air was 98%. His repeat chest x-ray is also shown below (Figure 27.2).

Figure 49.1: Chest x-ray

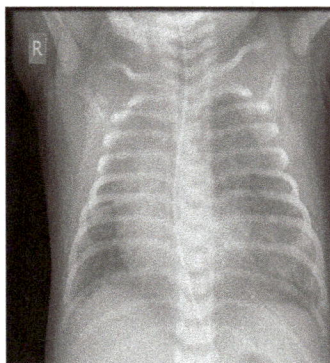

Figure 49.2: Chest x-ray

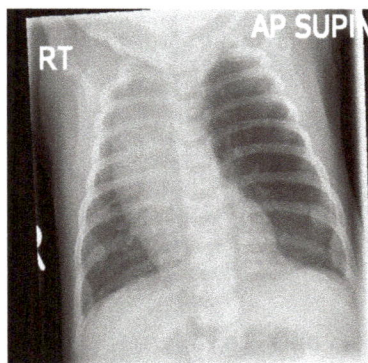

Q1. What is the most likely diagnosis?

Select <u>one</u> answer only

A. Congenital cystic adenomatoid malformation (CCAM) of the left lung
B. Congenital lobar emphysema (CLE) of the left lung
C. Foreign body inhalation
D. Left pneumothorax
E. Right upper lobe collapse/consolidation

Q2. How will you confirm the underlying diagnosis?

Select <u>one</u> answer only

A. Angiography of thoracic aorta
B. Bronchoscopy
C. CT of the chest
D. Echocardiography
E. Transillumination of the chest

Answer and Rationale

Q1.   **B: Congenital lobar emphysema (CLE) of left lung**
Q2.   **C: CT of the chest**

Congenital lobar emphysema (CLE) is a rare pathology characterised by overdistension of 1 or more lobes of the histologically normal lung. It is a heterogeneous disorder with disturbed lung growth, causing alteration in the airway or in the number or size of the alveoli. The overall incidence is reported to be 1 in 70,000 to 1 in 90,000 live births.

A clue can be ascertained from the site of any abnormality. The most commonly affected lobe is the left upper lobe (42%) followed by right middle (35%) or upper (21%) lobes, and it can be bilateral (20%). Aetiology is unknown in almost half of the cases, but various intrinsic and extrinsic factors have been described in the pathogenesis of CLE (1). It may be caused by abnormalities of the bronchial cartilage (reduced or absent bronchial cartilage resulting in intrinsic bronchial narrowing and bronchomalacia) or external bronchial compression from various causes (abnormal vessels, lymph nodes, cysts) resulting in air trapping, overdistension and emphysema.

Infants with CLE can present with respiratory symptoms soon after birth, but more commonly they present to clinicians after 1 to 2 months of age. Some infants are diagnosed incidentally when a chest x-ray is performed for another reason. Respiratory distress can often be accompanied by wheezing. The severity of symptoms depends upon the degree of over-inflation of the affected lobe, compression of the adjacent lung tissue and the resultant mediastinal shift produced by the ball-valve effect. The infant mostly presents with rapid respiratory rate, tachycardia, and chest retractions, which can worsen with increasing gas trapping in the emphysematous lobe and occasionally progresses into respiratory distress and respiratory failure. Other physical signs include decreased breath sounds over the affected lobe and the shift of the apical heartbeat to the opposite side of the chest, which makes clinicians consider the diagnosis of dextrocardia.

Some infants present following a surgical intervention as anaesthesia may precipitate acute hyperinflation of the lobe.

Despite advances in technology, pitfalls in diagnosis and management are not uncommon (2). The initial x-ray chest may not show the typical appearance of a hyperinflated lobe and may present with a region of increased density rather than hyperlucency, which can be mistaken for pneumonia. Similarly, CLE can sometimes be misdiagnosed as cystic malformation of the lung or even pneumothorax. In the latter situation, inappropriate placement of a chest drain may make the clinical situation even worse. The two can be differentiated radiologically by the presence of bronchovascular and alveolar markings within the emphysematous lobe. Sometimes, mucus plugging of the airway, a foreign body or inflammatory exudates can cause partial bronchial obstruction and distal hyperinflation (air trapping), giving a similar radiological appearance to CLE.

The correct diagnosis depends on a high level of clinical suspicion. The chest x-ray is helpful but not always diagnostic. A CT scan or MRI provides the most useful diagnostic information (3). A ventilation perfusion scan (V/Q scan) shows reduced perfusion of the affected lobe due to vessel compression and increased perfusion of normal lobes due to shunting. A bronchoscopy may be useful in older children in whom a foreign body must be ruled out. CLE may be diagnosed when respiratory distress occurs after birth, but the routine use of prenatal ultrasonography has resulted in prenatal diagnosis in some cases (4, 5). A precise prenatal diagnosis of CLE is difficult, however, because the increased echogenicity of the lungs is often too subtle to be appreciated in utero.

If clinically suspected, the patient should be discussed with the paediatric respiratory team and the plan for further management created. The treatment mainly depends upon the severity of the symptoms. The milder cases can be managed conservatively, but surgical resection of the emphysematous lobe may be indicated for severe cases.

Syllabus Mapping

Neonatology

- Be able to assess, diagnose and manage neonatal respiratory disorders with appropriate referral

- Be able to assess, diagnose and manage congenital anomalies presenting in the neonatal period and make appropriate referral

- Be able to assess, diagnose and manage neonatal surgical problems and make appropriate referral, including NEC

References and Further Reading

1. Berlinger NT, Porto DP, Thompson TR. Infantile lobar emphysema. Ann Otol Rhinol Laryngol 1987; 96: 106–111.

2. Tempe DK, Virmani S, Javetkar S, Banerjee A, Puri SK, Datt V. Congenital lobar emphysema: Pitfalls and management. Ann Card Anaesth 2010; 13: 53–58.

3. Stigers KB, Woodriing JH, Kanga JF. The clinical and imaging spectrum of findings in patients with congenital lobar emphysema. Pediatr Pulmonol 1992; 14: 160–170.

4. Olutoye OO, Coleman BG, Hubbard AM, Adzick NS. Prenatal diagnosis and management of congenital lobar emphysema. J Pediatr Surg 2000; 35: 792–795.

5. Quinton AE, Smoleniec JS. Congenital lobar emphysema. The disappearing chest mass: Antenatal ultrasound appearance. Ultrasound Obstet Gynecol 2001; 17: 169–171.

Chapter 49: A boy who can't play football
Dr Joanna Walker

A 7 year old, previously healthy, boy presents to the paediatric outpatient clinic with a 6 month history of lethargy, weakness, intermittent nausea and vomiting, and "feeling dizzy" when he stands up. He is no longer able to play a full game of football due to exhaustion. On examination, he is a generally healthy prepubertal boy and the systems examination is normal. His height is on the 50th centile, which is appropriate for the family size, and his weight is on the 9th centile. Supine blood pressure is 70/46 mmHg and erect blood pressure is 68/42 mmHg.

Investigations

Blood

Sodium	131 mmol/l
Potassium	5.3 mmol/l
Urea	8.2 mmol/l
Creatinine	25 μmol/l
Bicarbonate	23 mmol/l
Full blood count	Normal
IgA anti-tissue transglutaminase antibodies	Negative

Q1. Which of the following is the most likely diagnosis?

Select <u>one</u> answer only

A.   Addison disease (primary adrenal insufficiency)
B.   Distal (type 1) renal tubular acidosis
C.   Hypopituitarism
D.   Pseudohypoaldosteronism (PHA) type 1A
E.   Psychogenic polydipsia

Q2. Which of the following would be the most useful diagnostic test?

Select <u>one</u> answer only

A.   Plasma aldosterone level
B.   Short ACTH (Synacthen) stimulation test
C.   Thyroid function tests
D.   Urine calcium to creatinine ratio
E.   Water deprivation test

Answers and Rationale

Q1.   A: Addison disease (primary adrenal insufficiency)
Q2.   B: Short ACTH (Synacthen) stimulation test

The answer to this question requires knowledge of electrolyte control. Hyponatraemia is either dilutional as in, for example, Syndrome of Inappropriate Antidiuretic Hormone (SIADH) production or due to excess sodium losses. The clue here is the potassium and, in the absence of renal failure, hyponatraemia and hyperkalaemia strongly suggest aldosterone deficiency or resistance as in the various forms of PHA. PHA type 1A can be excluded because it presents in infancy with poor weight gain and severe hyperkalaemia, or presents transiently in infants with urosepsis often associated with dysplastic kidneys or urinary tract anomalies (1).

In distal (type 1) renal tubular acidosis (dRTA), the primary defect is a failure of acid secretion by the alpha intercalated cells of the cortical collecting duct of the distal nephron. There is associated sodium loss and the resulting vasoconstriction causes a compensatory increase in aldosterone. Aldosterone raises body sodium by increasing sodium reabsorption and potassium loss in the renal collecting ducts, so dRTA is characterised by metabolic acidosis and hypokalaemia. Patients sometimes present with associated weakness or with nephrocalcinosis due to hypercalciuria. This diagnosis can be discounted and, with it, the urine calcium to creatinine ratio.

Unlike the glucocorticoids (e.g. cortisol), aldosterone production is under renal control (not pituitary) in conjunction with the renin-angiotensin system. The glucocorticoids do have weak mineralocorticoid activity, but not to the extent that their deficiency due to pituitary failure would cause this electrolyte disturbance. Hypoglycaemia is the most common feature of hypopituitarism in infancy, but during childhood, it almost always presents with short stature and growth failure due to growth hormone deficiency. Thyroid function tests would then be important, although not diagnostic.

The electrolytes in psychogenic polydipsia are usually normal, but there may be mild – or rarely, moderate to severe – hyponatraemia but not the hyperkalaemia and the evidence of vasoconstriction with the elevated urea seen here. This answer and a water deprivation test can be excluded, although note that the latter is a potentially dangerous procedure and should only be performed by experienced personnel.

The likeliest diagnosis is primary adrenal failure (Addison disease) (1). Adrenal failure describes a situation where there is a deficient production of glucocorticoids and, often, mineralocorticoids. It is a life-threatening disorder caused by primary adrenal failure (Addison disease), inborn errors of steroid production (as in congenital adrenal hyperplasia) or secondary to ACTH deficiency as the result of an impairment in the hypothalamic-pituitary-adrenal axis.

Primary adrenal failure is most commonly the result of an autoimmune-mediated adrenalitis, when 21-hydroxylase antibodies are usually positive or, much more rarely, tuberculosis (TB). Presenting symptoms are often vague and include easy fatiguability, muscle weakness, nausea, anorexia and abdominal pain. Hyperpigmentation due to pituitary beta-lipoprotein secretion may be seen in the buccal mucosa, palmar creases, nipple areas, old scars or as a permanently "suntanned" appearance. Any postural hypotension is due to salt wasting.

The best, usually diagnostic, test of adrenal function is the short ACTH (Synacthen) test, although the dose of Synacthen in children and the definition of a normal response is controversial (2) and a paediatric endocrinologist must be consulted. Unless there is an unequivocally poor response, the short ACTH test is only part of the diagnostic pathway. An ACTH is taken at baseline and will be markedly elevated in Addison disease. Renin is the best biochemical estimate of overall body sodium and, therefore, of mineralocorticoid deficiency; thus, it is high in Addison disease. If it is measured, aldosterone may even be in the expected reference range but, nevertheless, it will be inappropriately low for the prevailing sodium.

A boy with primary adrenal failure should have adrenoleukodystrophy (ALD) – excluded because early treatment significantly alters the prognosis. ALD is the most common of the peroxisomal fatty acid beta-oxidation defects that result in the accumulation of very long chain fatty acids in all tissues. It is caused by mutations in ABCD1 and is X-linked, but is hugely heterogeneous with poor genotype to phenotype correlation, even within the same kindred. Two-thirds present in a severe childhood cerebral form, but other forms vary in terms of onset and clinical severity, ranging from adrenal insufficiency to progressive paraparesis (adrenomyeloneuropathy) in early adulthood.

Treatment of Addison disease is lifelong and involves replacement therapy with hydrocortisone (6–10 mg/m^2 per day) in 3 divided doses to mimic the diurnal rhythm and, almost always, fludrocortisone (0.1–0.15 mg/m^2 per day). Families (and their professionals) should have written instructions that state that doses of hydrocortisone must be at least doubled at times of physiological risk and given parenterally if necessary. They must also have open, immediate access to emergency facilities and, as the children get older and more independent, they should wear a warning talisman.

Syllabus Mapping

Endocrinology and Growth

- Be able to assess, diagnose and manage disorders of the adrenal, thyroid and parathyroid glands

Nephro-urology

- Demonstrate understanding, knowledge and management of fluid and electrolyte disturbance

References and Further Reading

1. Raine JE, Donaldson MDC, Gregory J, Van-Vliet G. Practical Endocrinology and Diabetes in Children, 3rd edition. Wiley-Blackwell, 2011. ISBN: 978-1-4051-9634-5.

2. Elder CJ, Sachdev P, Wright NP. The short Synacthen test: A questionnaire survey of current usage. Arch Dis Child 2012; 97(10): 870-3.

Chapter 50: HIV in pregnancy
Dr Lucy Hinds

A mother who is living in the UK is known to be HIV positive and has been on antiretroviral therapy throughout her pregnancy. At 37 weeks of gestation, her viral load is 184,000 copies/ml and she goes into labour.

Q1. Which of the following is the most appropriate management?

Select <u>one</u> answer only

A. Allow the mother to deliver vaginally and start the baby on single antiretroviral therapy
B. Allow the mother to deliver vaginally and start the baby on triple antiretroviral therapy
C. Deliver the baby by emergency Caesarean section and start the baby on single antiretroviral therapy
D. Deliver the baby by emergency Caesarean section and start the baby on triple antiretroviral therapy
E. Expedite vaginal delivery by the use of forceps and start the baby on single antiretroviral therapy

Q2. Which of the following is the currently recommended feeding regime most likely to reduce the transmission of HIV to this baby?

Select <u>one</u> answer only

A. Breastfeeding complemented by formula feeds
B. Breast milk bank feeds complemented by formula feeds
C. Exclusive breastfeeding
D. Exclusive formula feeding
E. Exclusive feeding with breast milk bank feeds

Answers and Rationale

Q1. **D: Deliver the baby by emergency Caesarean section and start the baby on triple antiretroviral therapy**

Q2. **D: Exclusive formula feeding**

Prevention of mother-to-child transmission has been one of the great successes in the fight against the global spread of HIV infection. Without intervention, the likelihood of vertical transmission is around 40%, with 10% of infants infected during pregnancy, 15% during delivery and 10–15% through breastfeeding. However, with appropriate clinical management, it is possible to reduce the risk of transmission to less than 2%. There are 3 points of intervention at which to prevent the transmission of the HIV virus from the mother to the child in the perinatal period, namely: the mode of delivery, the use of antiretroviral drugs and the method of feeding. Good communication between the obstetric and paediatric teams is essential. Whenever possible, a treatment plan should be put in place prior to the onset of labour and usually by 36 weeks of gestation. The planned management of an infant born to a mother with HIV infection is dependent on the mother's viral load throughout pregnancy and specifically at 36 weeks of gestation.

One of the most important factors in the prevention of mother-to-child transmission is the mode of delivery. If the mother has an undetectable viral load (<50 copies/ml) at 36 weeks of gestation, guidelines published by the British HIV Association (BHIVA) (1) recommend planned vaginal delivery, starting the baby on a 4-week course of zidovudine monotherapy within 48–72 hours of birth with advice to exclusively formula feed the baby. In this case, the mother's viral load is very high, which may be due to poor adherence with antiretroviral medication or the development of viral resistance. Whatever the cause, a detectable virus puts the baby at high risk of maternally transmitted disease. Thus, there is a need to maximise intervention. The BIHVA guidelines state that when the maternal load is >400 copies/ml at 36 weeks, a planned Caesarean section is recommended. These guidelines also state that for mothers with any detectable viral load (>50 copies/ml) at 36 weeks of gestation, the recommendation is for the infant to receive combination post-exposure prophylaxis with 3 drugs for 4 weeks (1).

Exclusive formula milk feeding is recommended for all mothers in the UK known to be HIV positive, regardless of antiretroviral therapy and infant post-exposure prophylaxis. Complete avoidance of breastfeeding removes the risk of postnatal transmission and is the current standard of care in the UK. This is in line with WHO guidance that exclusive feeding with infant formula should be recommended for women with HIV where it is affordable, feasible, acceptable and safe (2). In developing countries, infants who are exclusively formula fed have a significant morbidity and mortality related to diarrhoea and malnutrition. In these countries, WHO recommends exclusive breastfeeding in conjunction with antiretroviral therapy for 6 months. In these circumstances, the mother-to-child transmission rate of HIV infection can be reduced to 2% at 6 months of age (3).

Infants born to HIV-positive mothers should be tested for the HIV infection soon after birth. Maternal antibodies to HIV will cross the placenta and are therefore not useful in confirming the transmission of the virus. Instead, PCR molecular techniques are used to detect HIV RNA or DNA in the infant's blood. This should be performed within the first 48 hours of life, 2 weeks after stopping infant prophylaxis

(6 weeks of age) and 2 months post cessation of infant prophylaxis (12 weeks of age). HIV antibody testing for seroconversion should be checked at 18 months of age, but maternal antibodies may still be detectable up to 2 years of age. Current management regimes have resulted in an ever-improving prognosis for affected individuals, even into adult life, especially in the UK (4).

Syllabus Mapping

Infection, Immunology and Allergy

- Be able to assess, diagnose and manage infections acquired in the UK and overseas including TB, HIV and know when to refer

References and Further Reading

1. De Ruiter A et al. British HIV Association guidelines for the management of HIV infection in pregnant women 2012 (2014 interim review). HIV 2014 Suppl; 4: 1–77.

2. World Health Organization. HIV and infant feeding: A guide for healthcare managers and supervisors. Geneva, 2003. http://int/nutrition/publications/HIV_IF_guide for healthcare.pdf.

3. WHO Guidelines on HIV and infant feeding 2010. www.who.int/maternal_child_adolescent / documents/97892159935/en.

4. Bamford A, Lyall H. Paediatric HIV grows up: Recent advances in perinatally acquired HIV. Arch Dis Child 2015; 100: 183–188.